D0297570

MICROBIOLOGY PROCEDURES

MICROBIOLOGY PROCEDURES

The Selection and Interpretation
of Current Tests for Physicians,
Nurses, and Paramedical
Personnel

By

ROSE M. MORGAN, M.S., M.T. (A.S.C.P.)
North Dakota State University
Fargo, North Dakota

and

DOROTHY SHIESL GOOD, M.S., M.T. (A.S.C.P.)
John F. Kennedy Community Hospital
Edison, New Jersey

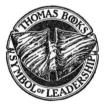

CHARLES C THOMAS · PUBLISHER
Springfield · Illinois · U.S.A.

Published and Distributed Throughout the World by
CHARLES C THOMAS • PUBLISHER
BANNERSTONE HOUSE
301-327 East Lawrence Avenue, Springfield, Illinois, U.S.A.

© *1973, by* CHARLES C THOMAS • PUBLISHER
ISBN 0-398-02471-5
Library of Congress Catalog Card Number: 70-198331

With THOMAS BOOKS *careful attention is given to all details of manufacturing and design. It is the Publisher's desire to present books that are satisfactory as to their physical qualities and artistic possibilities and appropriate for their particular use.* THOMAS BOOKS *will be true to those laws of quality that assure a good name and good will.*

Printed in the United States of America
N-1

PREFACE

Our book on clinical microbiology includes sections on bacteriology, virology, rickettsiology, mycology, and parasitology, and it has been prepared primarily as a general guide to the selection and interpretation of current laboratory procedures. It is not intended as a laboratory manual, and the details of technique are summarized only briefly under *Principle of the Test* for each procedure. The list of synonyms was devised with the intent of including all reasonable abbreviations by which the test is known. If any synonyms have been omitted, it is because the authors feel their similarity to other test synonyms might result in erroneous interpretations.

Proper identification of pathogens is of prime importance to the clinical microbiologist. In order to be of prime service, the microbiologist must be aware of the kind of specimen submitted and the need for the desired test. In this book, identification of an organism has been described in terms of methods available: culture on ordinary and differential media, routine and special stains, and biochemical tests.

There is no test more accurate than the manner in which the specimen is collected and handled. For this reason, the authors have emphasized the type of specimen needed, the quantity of such, instructions concerning preparation of the patient, preservatives used for specimens, and the proper handling of each test sample. The instructions concerning the kind and amount of the specimen required for the various procedures are those in general which we believe are predominately used in laboratories today. However, many laboratories have adapted their methods to the use of *micro* techniques, which are especially useful in pediatric medicine. Specific instructions for each laboratory should be carefully delineated and rigidly followed.

In noting the length of time required to perform each test, one must realize that the time listed is the time involved from the inauguration of the test to its completion. For example, a test such as a bacterial culture may require only 30 minutes of *actual working time,* but we have usually stated that "a minimum of 24 hours should be allowed for completion," since a long standing period is required for proper growth.

Because of the large number of terms used which may be unfamiliar to a number of readers, a glossary has been included. Wherever possible, photomicrographs have been incorporated with the purpose of enhancing comprehension of manifold procedures.

A number of individuals contributed generously to this book with their time and suggestions, and the authors wish to express their appreciation to these persons.

For their complete review of the manuscript: Robert D. Story, M.D., and Ronald Olin, M.D., both associated with the Department of Internal Medicine, Fargo Clinic, Fargo, North Dakota.

Significant contributions and advice were received from John D. LeMar, M.D., and James H. Coffey, M.D., both of the Department of Pathology, Fargo Clinic; Robert P. Bushell, M.D., Department of Obstetrics and Gynecology; Robert R. Ivers, M.D., Chairman, Department of Neurology, The Neuropsychiatric Institute; Laurence G. Pray, M.D., formerly with the Department of Pediatrics; Lester D. Shook, M.D., formerly with The Neuropsychiatric Institute; Henry G. Schriever, M.D., Director of Pathology, John F. Kennedy Community Hospital, Edison, New Jersey; Mrs. Marilyn Bronken, B.S., M.T. (ASCP), Chief Technologist, Fargo Clinic Laboratory; George L. Ulmer, B.S., M.T. (ASCP), Teaching Supervisor and Chief Microbiologist, Fargo Clinic; and Maxine J. Vestre, R.N., Instructor in Fundamentals and Medical Surgical I, Trinity Hospital, Minot, North Dakota.

Appreciation is sincerely expressed to Bonnie Silta, B.S., M.T. (ASCP) Barbara Swanson Hofer, B.S., M.T. (ASCP) and Carolyn Hass Paulus, B.S., M.T. (ASCP), for countless hours spent in proofreading this book.

ROSE MORGAN
DOROTHY GOOD

CONTENTS

SECTION II
MYCOLOGY

SECTION III
VIROLOGY

SECTION IV
RICKETTSIOLOGY

SECTION V
CLINICAL PARASITOLOGY

MICROBIOLOGY PROCEDURES

SECTION I

CLINICAL BACTERIOLOGY

ABSCESS CULTURE

The following materials should be collected for the procedure:

Sterile test tube.

Sterile swabs (two).

Sterile saline.

Sterile sponges.

Sterile scalpel blade.

Iodine or alcohol.

Procedure:

1. Cleanse the area surrounding the abscess with a sterile swab moistened with sterile saline. Wipe dry the site of the incision. Disinfect the area with an antiseptic, such as alcohol or iodine.

2. The medical doctor incises the abscess with a small, sterile blade if spontaneous rupture has not occurred.

3. Wipe away the first small quantity of pus with a sterile sponge.

4. Gently touch a sterile swab to the pus in the abscess, taking care not to infect the healthy tissue surrounding the abscess. In suspected cases of anthrax, special precaution must be taken in obtaining the specimen. In possible cases of tularemia, the material should be obtained either by biopsy or needle aspiration.

5. Label the specimen with the patient's name, room number, date, and exact time of collection. On the laboratory request-slip, report any antibiotic or chemotherapy which has been administered to the patient.

6. Transport the specimen to the laboratory immediately. Failure to do so may result in an unsatisfactory bacteriological examination, since certain pathogens are very fragile and tend to die under adverse conditions.

Principle of the Test:

Material from an abscess is cultured in an attempt to isolate any pathogenic organisms which may be present. The swab containing the material is used to inoculate the differential plate media (see *Culture, Routine,* p. 36), and the clock-streak method of isolation is used. The differential media most often used for the isolation of pathogens from an abscess are blood agar, eosin methylene blue agar, Staph 110, chocolate agar, thioglycollate broth, and glucose broth. Other media may be used, depending upon the suspected organism. If tuberculosis is suspected, some of the material may be inoculated onto Petragnani or Lowenstein's media. If mycotic structures are evident, part of the material should be inoculated on a Sabouraud dextrose agar slant and two mycosel slants.

SPECIMEN REQUIRED: Refer to *Nurses' Responsibility.*

PRESERVATIVE: None is permitted.

LENGTH OF TIME REQUIRED TO PERFORM TEST:

A minimum of 24 to 48 hours should be allowed for completion.

NORMAL VALUES: No pathogens isolated.

ABNORMAL FINDINGS:

Pathogens that may be isolated from an abscess include *Actinomyces, Bacillus anthracis, Clostridium* spp., *Corynebacterium* sp., *Mycobacterium tuberculosis, Neisseria gonorrhoeae, Pasteurella tularensis, Proteus* spp., *Staphylococcus aureus* (coagulase positive), *Streptococcus pyogenes, Treponema pallidum,* others.

ACID - FAST STAINING PROCEDURE

Ziehl-Neelsen Method for Acid-fast Organisms, Spengler's Method for Acid-fast Organisms, Acid-and-Alcohol Fast Stain, Kinyoun Stain for Acid-fast Organisms.

Nurses' Responsibility:

No special preparation of the patient is needed.

Principle of the Test:

Certain members of the genus *Mycobacterium,* and a few other bacteria, are resistant to decolorization by agents such as acid alcohol; because of this resistance to decolorization, they are termed "acid-fast." Acid-fast organisms stain red; other bacteria stain blue. The property of being acid-fast has been attributed to the fatty substances of the bacterial cell.

Procedure:

1. Flood the smear with carbolfuchsin solution and steam gently for three to five minutes. Care must be taken *not* to boil the stain. Renewal of the stain will prevent drying.

2. Wash the slide with tap water to remove the excess stain.

3. Decolorize the slide with acid-alcohol until the smear is colorless.

4. Wash with tap water.

5. Counterstain with methylene blue for approximately 15 to 30 seconds.

6. Wash with tap water and blot dry.

An *alternate* method is the *Spengler Method* as follows:

Procedure:

1. Flood the slide with carbolfuchsin solution, and steam gently for three to five minutes.

2. Tip the slide to remove the carbolfuchsin and apply picric acid alcohol for approximately three seconds.

3. Add four drops of 15% nitric acid for five seconds.

4. Pour off the nitric acid and apply picric acid alcohol until the slide appears yellow.

5. Wash with tap water.

This method is highly recommended for colorblind people, since acid-fast organisms stain black on a yellow background.

Another method is that of *Kinyoun*. This employs basic fuchsin, phenol, ethyl alcohol, and distilled water. The test is performed in much the same manner as the Ziehl-Neelson technique; however, no heat is necessary.

Currently, fluorescent antibody methods (see p. 52) for acid-fast organisms are being utilized with a high degree of accuracy. This technique employs auramine or rhodamine as the stain. Acid-fast organisms fluoresce with an orange-red color against a dark background.

The National Tuberculosis Association has outlined the method of reporting as follows:

Negative: No acid-fast bacilli found.

Rare: 1 to 2 acid-fast bacilli found in the entire smear.

Few: 3 to 9 acid-fast bacilli found in the entire smear.

Numerous: 10 or more acid-fast bacilli found in the entire smear.

SPECIMEN REQUIRED:

A few bacterial colonies of a 3 to 6 week culture, or a direct smear from tissues, urine, sputum, or cerebrospinal fluid.

PRESERVATIVE: None is required.

LENGTH OF TIME REQUIRED TO PERFORM TEST:

Allow 30 minutes following smear preparation.

NORMAL VALUES: No pathogenic acid-fast organisms found.

PATHOGENIC FINDINGS:

Mycobacterium tuberculosis, M. leprae, Actinomyces, Clostridium spp. (some) , *Nocardia asteroides,* few others.

ANIMAL INOCULATION

Synonym: Animal Injection.

Nurses' Responsibility:

No special preparation of the patient is needed.

Principle of the Test:

Certain diagnostic procedures may require the use of animals. Animal inoculation is of extreme value in the isolation and study of numerous microorganisms. Animals may be used for the propagation of viruses and bacteria, isolation of various bacteria in a pure culture, virulence and pathogenicity testing, preparation of autogenous vaccines, preparation of serological materials and immune sera, and numerous other procedures.

Many kinds of animals are currently being used in various research projects. Among these are the rabbit, hamster, guinea pig, mouse, rat, sheep, pig, cow, and chinchilla.

The animal is usually fastened into position by use of a restrainer. If necessary, the hair of the animal is clipped, and an antiseptic solution is applied to the area of the proposed injection. The animal should be made as comfortable as possible. The injection should be made by a person experienced in the inoculation of animals, in order to avoid excessive trauma. After the injection of the material, the animal is "tagged" by means of a small aluminum tag or by some other means for identification and is kept under close observation until death or evidence of disease.

Various methods of injection may be used. Routes of injection which are currently used include the following:

Subcutaneous: The skin of the animal is gently pinched between the thumb and forefinger until a fold is obtained. The hypodermic needle is pushed into the fold and to the subcutaneous layers of the skin while the material is injected.

Intravenous: This is most often the route chosen for injection of rabbits and frequently for guinea pigs. The ear or other selected site is shaven and the site exposed. The vein may be rubbed in order to dilate it. The material is injected directly into the vein. An inoculation box may be useful when injecting

9

rabbits and guinea pigs. For the injection of mice or rats, the tail vein is most often used. A cylinder of perforated zinc, which is closed with a V-wedged cork at one end and allows the tail to pass through, may be used.

Intramuscular: This route of injection is relatively simple and is frequently used. The material is injected into the thigh muscles.

Intracerebral: The animal is most often anesthetized during the injection. An incision may be made through the skin over the vertex for larger animals. A hole is drilled through the bone by means of a trephine, and the desired material is injected through the hole; the hole is then sutured with catgut. In smaller animals such as mice, trephining is not necessary. Rather, the mouse is anesthetized and the injection made directly through the skull.

Intracardial: The animal is first anesthetized and the anterior thorax shaved. The hypodermic needle is inserted to the left of the sternum, through the third intercostal space, and into the heart where the material is injected.

Intraperitoneal: This is a frequently used route of injection. The animal is usually held with its head down and the material injected into the midline of the lower half of the abdomen.

Other routes of injection include subdural, testicular, and intraocular.

SPECIMEN REQUIRED:
Serum, plasma, whole blood, urine, tissue, and bacterial cultures are commonly used. The material to be used will depend largely upon the diagnostician's needs.

PRESERVATIVE: Usually none is permitted.

LENGTH OF TIME REQUIRED TO PERFORM TEST:
No definite time can be ascertained, since each individual case reacts in a different way.

NORMAL VALUES: No pathogens found.

ABNORMAL FINDINGS:

Some of the pathogens which may be identified by this means are adenoviruses, *Blastomyces dermatiditis, Brucella abortus,* CCA viruses, *Clostridium tetani, Coccidioides immitis, Corynebacterium diphtheriae, Cryptococcus neoformans,* Coxsackie viruses A and B, ECHO viruses, EMC viruses, *Histoplasma capsulatum, Listeria monocytogenes, Mycobacterium tuberculosis,* para influenzal viruses, poliovirus, rabies virus.

AUTOGENOUS VACCINE

NURSES' RESPONSIBILITY:

No special preparation of the patient is needed.

PRINCIPLE OF THE TEST:

It is often necessary for a patient to be vaccinated against an organism with which he is frequently infected. This is done by preparing a vaccine from the lesion itself.

Procedure:

1. Select the desired media on which the bacteria are best suited to grow, and inoculate with the scrapings from the lesion. Blood agar or brain-heart infusion slants are frequently used.

2. Incubate the slants for 24 to 48 hours, or longer, depending upon the desired growth. The organism *must* be in pure culture.

3. Identify the isolated organism by Gram stain (p. 59), fluorescent antibody (p. 52), and biochemical tests necessary.

4. Transfer 5 ml of sterile phenol-saline solution to the surface of the slants containing the bacterial growth. The *entire* surface of the slant must be covered.

5. Loosen the bacterial growth from the surface by means of a sterilized nichrome or platinum loop. This allows the viable bacteria to be suspended in the phenol-saline solution.

6. Using sterile precautions, transfer the bacterial suspension into a Kolle flask and stopper.

7. Allow the flask to shake on a mechanical rotator for five to ten minutes or if manually, for at least 30 minutes or until all clumps of bacteria are dispersed and an even suspension is evident. Sterile beads in the flask may aid in the dispersion of the bacterial clumps.

8. Place the suspension of bacteria in a water bath at 65°C for 60 minutes to kill the bacteria. Formalin-phenol may at times be used rather than heating. Ultraviolet light has frequently been used.

9. Check for sterility by inoculating fluid thioglycollate and a blood agar or brain-heart infusion agar plate.

10. Incubate for 48 to 72 hours and observe for any growth.

If growth due to contamination has occurred, the vaccine must be discarded and the procedure repeated. If no growth occurs, the vaccine may be diluted and standardized by means of McFarland nephelometer standards until ready for use. Most vaccines are prepared so that the number of organisms given at one injection ranges from 100,000,000 to 1,000,000,000.

Numerous other procedures are currently available for the production of autogenous vaccines.

SPECIMEN REQUIRED:

Scrapings or a smear from the patient's lesion are needed.

PRESERVATIVE:

None can be used. The media must be inoculated immediately. LENGTH OF TIME REQUIRED TO PREPARE VACCINE: Allow five to eight days.

BACTERIA — NOMENCLATURE

Certain bacteria are known to clinicians by various terminology. The following is a listing of the preferred names of the various bacteria, as well as some of the most commonly known synonyms.

BACTERIA—PREFERRED NAMES AND SYNONYMS

PREFERRED NAME:	SYNONYM(S):
Actinobacillus actinomycetemcomitans	*Bacterium actinomycetem comitans, B. comitans.*
Actinobacillus mallei	*Bacillus mallei*, Glander's bacillus, *Malleomyces mallei, Pfeifferella mallei.*
Actinomyces israelii	*A. israeli, Streptothrix israeli.*
Aerobacter aerogenes	*Bacillus aerogenes, Bacterium aerogenes, B. lactis aerogenes.*
Aerobacter cloacae	*Bacillus cloacae, Bacterium cloacae.*
Alcaligenes faecalis	*Bacillus faecalis alcaligenes, Bacterium alcaligenes.*
Bacillus anthracis	*Anthrax bacillus, Davaine's bacillus.*
Bacteroides fragilis	*Bacillus fragilis, Ristella fragilis.*
Bordetella bronchiseptica	*Alcaligenes bronchisepticus, Bacillus bronchicanis, B. bronchisepticus, Bacterium bronchisepticus, Brucella bronchiseptica, Hemophilus bronchisepticus*
Borrelia novyi	*Spirochaeta novyi.*
Bordetella parapertussis	*Bacillus parapertussis, Hemophilus parapertussis.*
Bordetella pertussis	Bordet-Gengou bacillus, *Hemophilus pertussis.*
Borrelia recurrentis	*Protomycetum recurrentis, Spiroschaudinnia recurrentis.*
Borrelia vincentii	*Spirochaeta vincenti.*
Brucella abortus	*Bacterium abortus, Bang's abortion bacillus.*
Brucella melitensis	*Micrococcus melitensis, Streptococcus melitensis.*
Brucella suis	*Bacillus abortus.*

14

Calymmatobacterium granulomatis	*Donovania granulomatis,* Donovan bodies, epithelial cell parasites.
Clostridium bifermentans	*Bacillus bifermentans, B. bifermentans sporogenes, C. sordelli, Sordelli's bacillus.*
Clostridium botulinum	*Bacillus botulinus.*
Clostridium histolyticum	*Bacillus histolyticus.*
Clostridium novyi	*Bacillus novyi, B. oedematis maligni No. II, B. oedematis thermophilus, Novy's bacillus.*
Clostridium perfringens	Achalme's bacillus, *Bacillus aerogenes capsulatus, B. emphysematosus, B. perfringens, B. phlegmones emphysematosae, B. welchii, C. welchii,* gas bacillus, Welch's bacillus.
Clostridium septicum	*Bacillus septicus,* Gnon-Sachs' bacillus, *Vibrio pasteurii.*
Clostridium sporogenes	*Bacillus sporogenes.*
Clostridium tetani	*Bacillus tetani,* Nicolaier's bacillus.
Corynebacterium acnes	*Bacillus acnes, B. parvus liquefaciens, C. liquefaciens, Propionibacterium acnes.*
Corynebacterium diphtheriae	*Bacillus diphtheriae, C. ulcerans,* Diphtheria bacillus, Klebs-Loeffler bacillus, Loeffler's bacillus.
Corynebacterium pseudodiphtheriticum	Hofmann's bacillus.
Corynebacterium pyogenes	*Bacillus liquefaciens pyogenes bovis, B. pyogenes.*
Diplococcus pneumoniae	Coccus lanceole, diplococcus, Frankel's bacillus, micrococcus of rabbit septicemia, pneumococcus.
Erysipelothrix insidiosa	*Bacillus insidiosus, E. erysipeloides, E. murisepticus, E. porci, E. rhusiopathial.*
Escherichia coli	*Bacillus coli, B. escherichii, Bacterium coli, B. coli commune,* coli bacillus, colon bacillus.
Escherichia freundii	*Bacterium freundii.*
Fusobacterium fusiforme	*Bacillus fusiformis, B. hastilis, Corynebacterium fusiforme, Fusiformis dentium, F. fusiformis, Fusobacterium plautivincenti,* Vincent's bacillus.

Gaffkya tetragena	*Micrococcus tetragenus.*
Hemophilus aegypticus	*Bacillus aegypticus, Bacterium aegyptiacum, H. conjunctivitidis,* Koch-Weeks bacillus, Week's bacillus.
Hemophilus ducreyi	*Bacillus ulceris cancrosi, Coccobacillus ducreyi,* Ducrey's bacillus.
Hemophilus haemolyticus	Pritchett-Stillman's bacillus X.
Hemophilus influenzae	*Bacterium influenzae,* influenza bacillus, Morax' Axenfeld bacillus, Pfeiffer's bacillus.
Hemophilus parainfluenzae	Para-influenza bacillus.
Klebsiella ozaenae	Abel's bacillus, *Bacillus mucosus ozaenae, B. ozaenae, Bacterium ozaenae.*
Klebsiella pneumoniae	*Bacillus pneumoniae, Bacterium pneumonie crouposae, Hyalococcus pneumoniae, K. crouposa,* Friedlander's bacillus, Neumann's bacillus, pneumobacillus.
Klebsiella rhinoscleromatis	Rhinoscleroma bacillus.
Lactobacillus acidophilus	*Bacillus bifidus communis, B. bifidis.*
Lactobacillus casei	*Bacillus casei, Caseobacterium vulgare, Streptobacterium casei.*
Lactobacillus lactis	*Bacillus lactis acidi, Thermobacterium lactis.*
Lactobacillus leichmannii	*Bacillus leichmanni I.*
Leptospira icterohaemorrhagiae	*Spirochaeta ictero-haemorrhagiae, S. icterohaemorrhagiae japonica.*
Listeria monocytogenes	*Bacterium monocytogenes.*
Moraxella lacunata	*Bacillus duplex, B. lacunatus, Bacterium conjunctivitidis, B. conjunctivitis, Diplobacillus moraxinfeld.*
Moraxella liquefaciens	*Diplobacillus liquefaciens.*
Mycobacterium bovis	bovine tubercle bacillus, *M. tuberculosis* typus *bovinus.*
Mycobacterium fortuitum	*M. giae, M. minetti.*
Mycobacterium leprae	*Bacillus leprae,* Hansen's bacillus, leprosy bacillus.
Mycobacterium tuberculosis	*Bacillus tuberculosis, Bacterium tuberculosis,* human tubercle bacillus, Koch's bacillus, Much's bacillus, *M. tuberculosis* var. *hominis.*

Mycoplasma hominis	*Micromyces hominis* (group I) .
Mycoplasma fermentans	*Micromyces hominins* (group II) .
Mycoplasma pneumoniae	Eaton agent, Eaton pleuropneumonia-like agent.
Neisseria catarrhalis	*Micrococcus catarrhalis.*
Neisseria gonorrhoeae	*Gonococcus neisseri, Micrococcus gonorrhoeae.*
Neisseria meningitidis	*Diplococcus intracellularis meningitidis, Micrococcus intracellularis, M. meningitidis, N. weichselbaumii,* meningococcus, Weichselbaum's bacillus.
Nocardia asteroides	*Cladothrix asteroides.*
Paracolobactrum aerogenoides	*Para-aerogenes.*
Paracolobactrum coliforme	*Para-coli.*
Paracolobactrum intermedium	*Para-freundii.*
Pasteurella multocida	*Bacillus septicaemiae haemorrhagicae, Bacterium multocidum, P. septica.*
Pasteurella pestis	*Bacterium pestis,* Kitasato's pestis, pest bacillus.
Pasteurella pseudotuberculosis	*Bacillus pseudotuberculosis, Streptobacillus pseudotuberculosis rodentium.*
Pasteurella tularensis	*Bacterium tularense.*
Peptococcus activus	*Staphylococcus activus.*
Peptococcus aerogenes	*Micrococcus aerogenes, staphylococcus aerogenes.*
Peptococcus anaerobius	Anaerobic staphylococcus *Micrococcus anaerobius, Staphylococcus anaerobius.*
Peptococcus asaccharolyticus	*Micrococcus asaccharolyticus, Staphylococcus asaccharolyticus.*
Peptococcus constellatus	*Diploccoccus constellatus.*
Peptococcus grigoroffii	*Micrococcus grigoroffi.*
Proteus inconstans	*Bacillus inconstans.*
Proteus mirabilis	*Bacterium mirabilis.*
Proteus morganii	*Bacillus morgani, Bacterium morgani, Salmonella morgani.*
Proteus rettgeri	*Bacterium rettgeri, P. entericus, Shigella rettgeri.*
Proteus vulgaris	*Bacterium vulgare.*

Pseudomonas aeruginosa	*Bacille pyocyanique, B. pyocyaneus, Bacterium aeruginosum,* blue pus organism, *P. pyocyanea.*
Pseudomonas pseudomallei	*Bacillus pseudomallei, B. whitmori, Loefflerella pseudomallei, Malleomyces pseudomallei,* Whitmore's bacillus.
Salmonella choleraesuis	*Bacterium cholerae suis, Pasteurella salmoni*
Salmonella enteritidis	*Bacillus enteritidis,* Gaertner's bacillus.
Salmonella hirschfeldii	*Bacillus paratyphosus B, B. paratyphosus C,* Hirschfeld's bacillus, Paratyphoid C bacillus.
Salmonella paratyphi	*Bacterium paratyphi, B. paratyphi A,* Paratyphoid A bacillus.
Salmonella schottmuelleri	*Bacillus paratyphi alcaligenes, B. schottmulleri, Bacterium paratyphi B,* Paratyphoid B bacillus.
Salmonella typhimurium	*Bacillus typhi murium,* Nocard's bacillus.
Salmonella typhosa	*B. typhi, B. typhi abdominalis, B. typhosus, Bacterium typhosum,* B. typhi Eberth's bacillus, Eberthella typhosa, *S. typhi,* Typhoid bacillus, Typhus Bacillen.
Shigella alkalescens	*Bacillus alkalescens, Proshigella alkalescens.*
Shigella dispar	*Bacillus ceylanensis B, B. dispar, Castellanus castellanii, Proshigella dispar.*
Shigella dysenteriae	*Bacillus dysenterae, B. shigae, S. shigae.*
Shigella flexneri	*Bacillus dysenteriae* Flexner, *B. dysenteriae* Shiga, *B. paradysenteriae,* Flexner's bacillus, pseudodysentery bacillus, *S. paradysenteriae,* Strong's bacillus.
Shigella sonnei	*Bacillus dispar, Bacterium sonnei,* Duval's bacillus, *Proshigella sonnei,* Sonne's bacillus.
Spirillum minus	*Spirochaeta muris.*
Staphyloccus aureus	*Micrococcus albus, M. aureus, M. citreus, M. pyogenes, S. albus, S. citreus, S. pyogenes albus, S. pyogenes aureus, S. pyogenes citreus.*

Staphylococcus epidermidis	*Albococcus epidermidis, Micrococcus epidermidis, S. epidermidis albus.*
Streptobacillus moniliformis	*Actinomyces muris, A. muris ratti, Asterococcus muris, Haverhillis moniliformis, Nocardia muris, Proactinomyces muris, Streptothrix muris ratti.*
Streptococcus agalactiae	Group B (Lancefield) Streptococcus, *S. mastitidis, S. nocardi.*
Streptococcus anginosus	Group F and Type I Group II (Lancefield) Streptococci, Minute hemolytic Streptococci.
Streptococcus bovis	Group D (Lancefield) Streptococcus.
Streptococcus equisimilis	Group C (Lancefield) Streptococcus; *S. pyogenes type B, S. pyogenes* humanus C.
Streptococcus faecalis	*Enterococcus, E. proteiformis,* Group D. (Lancefield) Streptococcus, *Micrococcus ovalis, S. ovalis.*
Streptococcus mitis	Groups N and O (Lancefield) Streptococcus, *S. viridans.*
Streptococcus pyogenes	Erysipelokokkus, Group A (Lancefield) Streptococcus, *Micrococcus scarlatinae, S. erysipelatos, S. hemolyticus, S. scarlatinae.*
Streptococcus salivarius	Group F (Lancefield) Streptococcus.
Streptococcus sanguis	Group H (Lancefield) Streptococcus, *S. hominis, S.* s.b.e.
Treponema carateum	*T. americanus, T. herrejoni, T. pictor, T. pintae.*
Treponema microdentium	Small oval treponema.
Treponema mucosum	*T. dentium.*
Treponema pallidum	*Spirochaete pallida.*
Veillonella alcalescens	*Micrococcus gazogenes, M. gazogenes alcalescens anaerobius, V. gazogenes.*
Veillonella discoides	*Neisseria discoides.*
Veillonella parvula	*Staphylococus parvulus.*
Veillonella reniformis	*Diplococcus reniformis, Micrococcus reniformis, Neisseria reniformis.*
Veillonella vulvovaginitidis	*Neisseria vulvovaginitis*

Microbiology Procedures

Vibrio comma Cholera vibrio, comma bacillus, *Micro-spira comma, Spirillum cholerae asiaticae, V. cholerae.*

BACTERIOLOGICAL CHEMICAL TESTS

Biochemical tests are often employed in the identification of various bacteria. Several of these tests are listed alphabetically throughout the book as follows:

Carbohydrate Fermentation Tests for Identification of Bacteria.
Catalase Test.
Citrate Utilization Test.
Coagulase Test.
Decarboxylase Test for Identification of Bacteria.
Gelatin Liquefaction by Bacteria.
Hydrogen Sulfide Test for Bacterial Identification.
Indole Test.
Methyl Red Test for Bacteria.
Motility Tests for Bacteria.
Nitrate Reduction Test.
Oxidase Test.
Phenylalanine Deaminase Test.
Potassium Cyanide Test for Bacterial Identification.
Urease Test.
Voges-Proskauer Test.

BLOOD CULTURE (BATTERY)

The physician will frequently order a battery of several blood cultures in an attempt to isolate a specific organism or organisms from the patient's blood. The battery often reveals the organism suspected, whereas a single culture may not. In various diseases, the possibility of isolating the pathogenic organisms will depend on the stage of the disease. For example, in infections such as anthrax or typhoid fever, the causative organisms may be found during the first few days of the illness but may disappear from the bloodstream during the later period.

Timing of blood culturing is also important. For example, in subacute bacterial endocarditis, the physician may order blood cultures at different intervals during the day, i.e. at 8 A.M., 12 noon, 4 P.M., and again at 8 P.M.; or, they may be performed every 24 hours for three or four consecutive days.

See also *Blood Culture (Single)*.

BLOOD CULTURE (SINGLE)

SYNONYM: Culture, Blood.

NURSES' RESPONSIBILITY:

1. Make certain the patient is made comfortable.

2. Close *all* windows in the room during the actual drawing of the blood sample, to avoid contamination.

3. Report on the laboratory request-slip any pertinent information such as antibiotic therapy so that the laboratory may add drug inhibitors to the culture if necessary. If an intravenous injection has been given six hours prior to the drawing of the sample, this should be reported. Report any thermal reaction along with the exact time at which it occurred.

4. A prep tray which includes the following should be set up:
Tourniquet.
Culture bottles.
Sterile syringes and needles.
Sterile gauze and sponges.
Forceps.
2% aqueous iodine.
80% isopropyl alcohol.

PRINCIPLE OF THE TEST:

Employing aseptic technique, the site of the venipuncture is prepared. The area of the selected vein, most often the median basilic vein of the arm, is swabbed with a 2% tincture of iodine solution using a saturated cotton-tipped swab. The solution is allowed to dry and is removed by rubbing with gauze sponges saturated with 80% isopropyl alcohol. A few milliliters of venous blood are drawn by sterile technique and are inoculated onto a select media. Most often the choice of media is a blood agar plate, thioglycollate broth, and a Castaneda bottle containing blood culture broth. Commercial sterile blood culture sets are available and are highly recommended. The medium most often consists of a bottle of broth (such as tryptone, heart infusion, or trypticase soy) for aerobic cultures, and a bottle of thioglycollate medium for anaerobic cultures. Other media may be used, depending upon the organism (s) suspected. The blood culture is subcultured on the second, fourth, seventh, and fourteenth days. These samples are most often cultured on a blood agar plate, eosin methylene blue, or MacConkey agar plate, and a Gram stain (see p. 59) is made. In the case of negative cultures, the culture is usually observed 10 to 14 days before a final report of "no growth" is given. Some diseases such as typhoid fever and brucellosis, however, require a much longer growth period and must be kept at least six weeks before a final negative result is reported.

The blood cultures are incubated aerobically at 37°C and also anaerobically in an anaerobic jar. The cultures are examined daily throughout the first week and at various times thereafter for evidence of bacterial growth.

Pathogenic organisms that may occur in the blood include. *Escherichia coli, Staphylococcus aureus, Neisseria meningitidis, N. gonorrhoeae, Diplococcus pneumoniae, Streptococcus viridans, Brucella* spp., *Salmonella typhosa, Histoplasma capsulatum, Hemophilus influenzae, Proteus* spp., *Clostridium* spp., *Pasteurella tularensis, Listeria monocytogenes, Herellea* spp., *Pseudomonas aeruginosa, Aerobacter aerogenes, Spirillum minus, Leptospira icterohaemorrhagiae,* others.

SPECIMEN REQUIRED:

Five cubic centimeters of venous blood are needed. Usually the specimen does not require an anticoagulant. However, if one is used, 2% sodium citrate is the choice.

PRESERVATIVE: None is required.

LENGTH OF TIME REQUIRED TO PERFORM TEST:

A minimum of 10 to 14 days is needed for most negative cultures and up to six weeks for others, depending upon the suspected organism (s) .

NORMAL VALUES: No organisms isolated.

MAY BE POSITIVE IN:

Brucellosis, influenza, meningitis, pneumonia, salmonellosis, septicemia, subacute bacterial endocarditis, typhoid fever.

CARBOHYDRATE FERMENTATION TESTS FOR IDENTIFCATION OF BACTERIA

SYNONYM: Sugar Fermentation Test for Bacterial Identification.

NURSES' RESPONSIBILITY:

No special preparation of the patient is needed.

PRINCIPLE OF THE TEST:

Certain bacteria react in various ways when in contact with a medium containing a specific carbohydrate. The usual media (primarily sugars) employed in fermentation studies are glucose, maltose, sucrose, lactose, salicin, mannitol, starch, galactose, dulcitol, glycerol, inulin, trehalose, mannose, rhamnose, raffinose, inosite, levulose, and xylose.

The medium is inoculated with the test colonies, incubated at 37°C for 8 to 24 hours, and observed for acid formation and gas production. This solid medium is most often inoculated by means of a straight needle containing a few of the test organisms, by plunging it deeply into the medium with a stabbing motion.

An alternate method employs a plate medium which uses small paper discs impregnated with various carbohydrates. The plates are incubated at 37°C, and preliminary examination is made at eight hours for the characteristic yellow zone indicating acidity, and for bubbles and/or splits in the agar due to production of gas.

A third method employs the fermentation tube method. This tube contains a fermentation sugar which is inoculated with the test organism (s) . One end of the tube is sealed off and placed in an inverted position within a larger tube of liquid medium. The sealed end emerges just above the level of the fluid. If there is gas production, it collects in the smaller tube and rises toward the sealed end. The fermentation tests are most frequently used in the diagnosis of the Enterobacteriaceae, although they may be used for identification of other bacteria.

SPECIMEN REQUIRED:

A few colonies of the test organism are needed.

PRESERVATIVE: None is permitted.

LENGTH OF TIME REQUIRED TO PERFORM TEST:

A minimum of 8 to 24 hours following the initial growth of the culture must be allowed.

SIGNIFICANCE OF FINDINGS: Refer to Table I.

TABLE I
FERMENTATION REACTIONS OF ENTEROBACTERIACEAE

	Adonitol	Amygdalin	Arabinose	Cellobiose	Dextrin	Dulcitol	Erythritol	Esculin	Fructose	Galactose	Glucose	Glycerol	Glycogen	Inulin	Inositol
Aerobacter aerogenes	V	—	AG	AG	AG	V	—	AG	AG	AG	AG	AG	—	V	AG
Escherichia freundii (Citrobacter)	V	NF	AG	V	NF	V	NF	V	AG	AG	AG	AG	NF	NF	V
Escherichia coli	V	—	AG	NF	NF	V	—	V	AG	AG	AG	V	—	V	—
Klebsiella pneumoniae	A	—	A	—	—	V	—	—	—	AG	AG	—	—	—	A
Paracolobactrum aerogenoides (Hafnia)	—	—	AG	AG	AG	—	—	AG	AG	AG	AG	AG	—	—	—
Paracolobactrum arizonae (Arizona)	NF	—	—	—	—	NF	—	—	—	—	AG	—	—	—	NF
Paracolobactrum coliforme	R	—	AG	AG	NF	V	—	V	AG	AG	AG	V	NF	R	NF
Paracolobactrum intermedium	V	NF	AG	AG	NF	V	NF	V	AG	AG	AG	AG	NF	NF	AG
Proteus inconstans (Providencia)	D	NF	NF	NF	NF	NF	NF	NF	NF	NF	AG	V	NF	NF	NF
Proteus mirabilis	—	—	—	—	NF	—	—	—	AG	AG	AG	—	—	—	NF

Organism																	
Proteus morganii	NF	—	NF	NF	—	—	—	NF	NF	—	—	AG	AG	AG	—	—	NF
Proteus rettgeri (Entericus)	AG	NF	—	—	A	—	—	—	—	—	—	AG	AG	AG	—	—	V
Proteus vulgaris	—	—	—	NF	—	—	—	NF	—	—	—	AG	AG	AG	—	—	—
Salmonella paratyphi A	NF	AG	—	D	—	—	—	—	—	—	—	AG	—	AG	—	—	NF
Salmonella typhosa	NF	D	—	D	—	—	—	—	—	—	—	A	—	A	—	—	V
Shigella alkalescens	—	—	—	A	NF	—	—	—	—	—	—	A	—	A	—	—	—
Shigella boydii	—	A	—	—	—	—	—	—	—	—	—	A	—	A	—	—	—
Shigella dysenteriae	NF	NF	—	NF	—	—	—	—	—	—	A	A	A	A	A	—	—
Shigella flexneri	NF	A	—	NF	—	—	—	—	—	—	—	A	—	A	—	—	—
Shigella sonnei	NF	A	—	NF	—	—	—	—	—	—	A	A	A	A	—	—	NF

KEY:

A = Acid
G = Gas
V = Variable

D = Delayed or slow
NF = Nonfermented
R = Rarely fermented

	Lactose	Maltose	Mannitol	Mannose	Melezitose	Pectin	Propectin	Raffinose	Rhamnose	Salicin	Sorbitol	Starch	Sucrose	Trehalose	Xylose
Aerobacter aerogenes	AG	AG	AG	—	—	—	NF	AG	—	AG	AG	AG	V	—	—
Escherichia freundii (Citrobacter)	AG	AG	AG	AG	NF	—	—	AG	AG	V	AG	—	V	AG	AG
Escherichia coli	AG	AG	AG	—	—	R	—	V	AG	V	—	—	V	—	AG
Klebsiella pneumoniae	AG	A	A	—	—	—	—	—	A	A	A	A	A	—	A
Paracolobactrum aerogenoides (Hafnia)	AG	AG	AG	—	—	—	—	AG	AG	AG	AG	A	A	—	—
Paracolobactrum arizonae (Arizona)	V	—	—	—	—	—	—	—	V	V	—	AG	NF	—	—
Paracolobactrum coliforme	AG	AG	AG	—	—	R	—	V	AG	V	—	NF	V	—	AG
Paracolobactrum intermedium	AG	AG	AG	AG	NF	—	—	AG	AG	V	AG	V	—	AG	AG
Proteus inconstans (Providencia)	NF	NF	NF	NF	NF	NF	NF	NF	NF	NF	NF	NF	D	NF	NF
Proteus mirabilis	NF	NF	NF	—	—	—	—	—	—	—	—	—	D	AG	AG

Organism															
Proteus morganii	NF	NF	AG	—	—	AG	—	—	NF	NF	—	AG	NF	NF	R
Proteus rettgeri (Entericus)	NF	NF	AG	—	—	—	—	V	V	—	—	—	D	—	—
Proteus vulgaris	NF	AG	NF	—	—	—	—	—	—	—	—	AG	AG	—	—
Salmononella paratyphi A	NF	AG	AG	NF	—	—	—	NF	AG	NF	—	—	NF	AG	NF
Salmonella typhosa	NF	A	A	—	—	—	—	NF	NF	NF	—	—	NF	A	V
Shigella alkadescens	NF	A	A	—	—	—	—	A	NF	NF	—	—	A	—	A
Shigella boydii	—	R	A	—	—	—	—	—	—	—	—	R	R	—	—
Shigella dysenteriae	—	NF	NF	—	—	—	A	NF	NF	—	—	—	NF	—	NF
Shigella flexneri	NF	A	A	—	—	—	—	A	NF	NF	—	—	A	—	V
Shigella sonnei	A	A	A	—	—	—	A	A	—	—	—	—	A	—	NF

CATALASE TEST

Nurses' Responsibility:

No special preparation of the patient is needed.

Principle of the Test:

Certain bacteria, which have an iron-porphyrin-containing enzyme known as *catalase*, decompose hydrogen peroxide to molecular oxygen and water. A drop of hydrogen peroxide is added to a bacterial suspension and the mixture is observed for visible bubbles of oxygen which indicate a positive test; no gas formation signifies a negative test.

Specimen Required:

A few colonies of an 18 to 24 hour bacterial culture which has not been grown on blood agar are needed.

Preservative: None is permitted.

Length of Time Required to Perform Test:

A minimum of 15 minutes following growth of the bacterial culture should be allowed.

Positive in:

Cultures from almost all aerobic bacteria and some facultative anaerobes, such as micrococci and staphylococci (some).

Negative in:

Cultures of clostridia, pneumococci, shigella, staphylococci (some), streptococci.

CEREBRAL SPINAL FLUID CULTURE

SYNONYM: Spinal Fluid Culture.

NURSES' RESPONSIBILITY:

Care *must* be taken to avoid contact of the spinal fluid with any disinfectants. All antibiotic therapy must be noted along with the request.

PRINCIPLE OF THE TEST:

A loopful of the sterile cerebrospinal fluid sediment is inoculated onto the culture medium best suited for the suspected organism (s) and the clock-streak method of isolation is used.

A highly recommended method of inoculation is to allow a few drops of the spinal fluid to flow directly from the lumbar puncture needle into preheated culture medium. The media of choice for isolation of organisms in cerebrospinal fluid most often includes a blood agar plate, glucose broth, a glucose agar slant, thioglycollate medium, and an eosin methylene blue plate. At times a chocolate agar plate may be used in the isolation of anaerobic organisms.

Another aid may include the addition of 5 ml of dextrose ascitic fluid semisolid agar to the spinal fluid sediment. This media has been shown to be highly effective in the isolation of causative agents of bacterial meningitis when plates and streak plates have been negative. The semisolid medium will become cloudy and yellow in appearance when growth is present. All cultures are inoculated and incubated under ordinary conditions, and some are placed in a candle jar at 37°C for 48 to 72 hours.

A direct Gram stain (see p. 59) and the Quellung reaction (see p. 81) are sometimes of diagnostic aid.

SPECIMEN REQUIRED:

A few drops of freshly drawn, clear cerebrospinal fluid are needed.

PRESERVATIVE:

None is permitted; however, the specimen must be cultured as soon as possible after it has been withdrawn. If it is not possible to do immediate culturing, the specimen must be incubated at 37°C until used.

LENGTH OF TIME REQUIRED TO PERFORM TEST:

A minimum of 24 to 48 hours must be allowed.

NORMAL VALUES: No organisms isolated.

SIGNIFICANCE OF FINDINGS:

Pathogenic bacteria which are most often isolated from the cerebrospinal fluid include *Diplococcus pneumoniae, Escherichia coli, Hemophilus influenzae, Leptospira* spp., *Listeria monocytogenes, Mycobacterium tuberculosis, Neisseria meningitidis, Pseudomonas aeruginosa, Proteus* spp., *Staphylococcus aureus, Streptococcus pyogenes.*

CITRATE UTILIZATION TEST

SYNONYM: Simmon's Citrate Utilization Test.

NURSES' RESPONSIBILITY:

Certain bacterial organisms, when in an ammonium salt medium, utilize sodium citrate as the chief source of carbon. The bacterial colonies are streaked onto a Simmon's citrate slant and the reaction observed after two hours. The test is considered part of the IMViC (indole methyl red Voges-Proskauer citrate) formula and is read as follows:

Prussian blue color on slant: Positive.

No change in slant (green color): Negative.

SPECIMEN REQUIRED: A few colonies of the test organism are needed.

PRESERVATIVE: None is permitted.

LENGTH OF TIME REQUIRED TO PERFORM TEST:

A minimum of two hours after previous growth of test organisms should be allowed.

NEGATIVE IN:

Escherichia coli, Shigella spp., few other bacteria.

POSITIVE IN:

Aerobacter aerogenes, Citrobacter freundii, Klebsiella pneumoniae, Hafnia spp., *Proteus* spp. (some) , *Providencia, Salmonella* spp., *Serratia marcescens,* few other bacteria.

COAGULASE TEST

SYNONYM: Staphylococcus Pathogenicity Test.

NURSES' RESPONSIBILITY:
No special preparation of the patient is needed.

PRINCIPLE OF THE TEST:
Pathogenic strains of *Staphylococcus* produce a substance known as prostaphylcoagulase which reacts with an activator, somewhat similar to prothrombin, to form the active clotting agent known as *coagulase*. Coagulase in turn reacts with fibrinogen to form fibrin; thus, the *Staphylococcus* is coagulated by human or rabbit oxalated or citrated plasma.

The test is used in distinguishing between pathogenic and nonpathogenic organisms. The ability of certain organisms to coagulate plasma is directly correlated with pathogenicity.

The test may be run either as a slide (rapid method) or test-tube method. One colony of an 18 to 24 hour culture of organisms is emulsified in a drop of sterile distilled water on a glass slide. One drop of a commercial lyophilized plasma is added and mixed thoroughly into the emulsion. Agglutination of the mixture occurs within 30 seconds if the test is positive. If the test is negative, the finding is confirmed by using the test-tube method which employs a three-hour incubation of the mixture at 37 °C. Since a small number of sera require a longer period of incubation, tubes which show no coagulation after three hours are incubated at 37° for 18 hours. A known positive *Staphylococcus* should be run as a control measure in conjunction with the test.

SPECIMEN REQUIRED:
One to three colonies of the test organism are needed.

PRESERVATIVE: None is permitted.

LENGTH OF TIME REQUIRED TO PERFORM TEST:
Slide Test: Allow one hour for completion.
Tube Test: Allow up to 18 hours for negative tests.

NORMAL VALUES: Negative.

POSITIVE IN:

Pathogenic, toxin-producing strains of *Staphylococcus,* such as *S. aureus.* Occasional strains of other bacteria may give a positive reaction. These include *Bacillus subtilis, Escherichia coli, Pseudomonas pyocyanea, Serratia marcescens.*

CULTURE (ROUTINE)

SYNONYM: Bacteriological Culture (Routine).

Although many different methods for bacteriological cultures are in use today, most microbiologists are in agreement with the following method. A small amount of the material (inoculum) to be cultured is placed on the edge of the differential plate media. A wire inoculating loop of platinum, nichrome, or other suitable material is used to spread this material on the plate. A clock-streak method is most often used to ensure isolation of the bacterial colonies, thus enabling easier identification of the organisms.

After the differential plates are streaked, the plates are incubated at 37°C in an inverted position and are observed for growth at 24 and 48 hours. In addition to the plate technique, many microbiologists use tubes of broth and thioglycollate media for identification of the organisms. Many other media are presently in use, but the most commonly used are blood agar, eosin methylene blue, Salmonella-Shigella agar, MacConkey's, Simmon's citrate, Selenite F, and Staph 110.

The reader is referred to the individual tests, listed alphabetically in this book as follows:

Abscess Culture.
Blood Culture.
Ear Culture.
Eye Culture.
Feces, Routine Culture for Bacteria.
Joint Fluid Culture.
Pleural Fluid Culture.
Sinus Culture.
Spinal Fluid Culture.
Sputum, Routine Culture.
Throat and Nose Culture.
Urine Culture (Qualitative and Quantitative).
Wound Culture.

DECARBOXYLASE TEST

SYNONYM:

Decarboxylation of Amino Acids for Identification of Bacteria.

NURSES' RESPONSIBILITY:

No special preparation of the patient is needed.

PRINCIPLE OF THE TEST:

Certain organisms have the ability to decarboxylate various amino acids. The test is most frequently employed in the differentiation of the Enterobacteriaceae but may also be used in the study of various other bacteria. The decarboxylation test most often employs lysine, arginine, or ornithine in the inoculated medium. The organism possessing a specific capacity has the ability to remove a carbon dioxide group from the amino acid, converting it to an amine.

SPECIMEN REQUIRED: A few colonies of the test organism are needed.

PRESERVATIVE: None is permitted.

LENGTH OF TIME REQUIRED TO PERFORM TEST:

A minimum of two to six hours should be allowed.

NORMAL VALUES: There are no set normal values for this test.

POSITIVE IN:

ARGININE	LYSINE	ORNITHINE
—	*Aerobacter* (subgroup B)	*Aerobacter* (subgroup A, B)
	Hafnia	*Hafnia*
	Klebsiella	*Klebsiella*
	Proteus (some species)	
		Proteus mirabilis
		Proteus morganii
	Serratia	*Serratia*

NEGATIVE IN:

ARGININE	LYSINE	ORNITHINE
Proteus (all species)	*Aerobacter* (subgroup A)	*Proteus vulgaris*
	Citrobacter	
	Proteus (some species)	*Proteus rettgeri*
		Providencia
	Shigella	

37

EAR CULTURE

NURSES' RESPONSIBILITY:

A prep tray which includes the following should be set up:

Sterile swabs in tubes.

Sterile sponges.

1% tincture iodine.

80% isopropyl alcohol.

Most otologists prefer to collect the material from an ear infection themselves. However, should the otologist request the nurse to obtain the specimen, the following procedure is recommended.

Procedure:

1. Cleanse the skin and external auditory canal with a 1% tincture of iodine solution. Follow by swabbing with an alcohol solution.

2. Obtain the pus by touching the surface of the infected area with a sterile swab.

3. Return the swab to the sterile tube from which it was taken.

4. Transport the specimen to the laboratory immediately after collection. Failure to do so may result in an unsatisfactory bacteriological examination, since certain pathogens are very fragile, need moisture, and tend to die under adverse conditions.

PRINCIPLE OF THE TEST:

Material from the auditory canal (or other parts of the ear) is cultured in an attempt to isolate any pathogenic organisms which may be present.

The swab containing the material is rubbed onto the differential plate media (see *Culture, Routine,* p. 36) and the clock-streak method of isolation is used. Cultures are usually made both aerobically and anaerobically. The differential media most often used in the isolation of pathogens from the ear are blood agar, eosin methylene blue, chocolate agar, MacConkey agar, thioglycollate medium, and brain-heart infusion agar. Cultures may also be made for fungal growth (see *Fungus Culture,* p. 129) if the physician deems it necessary.

SPECIMEN REQURIED: See *Nurses' Responsibility.*

PRESERVATIVE: None is permitted.

LENGTH OF TIME REQUIRED TO PERFORM TEST:
A minimum of 24 to 48 hours should be allowed.

NORMAL VALUES: No pathogens isolated.

ABNORMAL FINDINGS:
Pathogens that may be isolated from ear cultures include alpha and beta hemolytic streptococci, anaerobic streptococci, *Aspergillus fumigatus, Candida albicans, Corynebacterium diphtheriae,* diphtheroids, *Diplococcus pneumoniae, Proteus* spp., *Pseudomonas aeruginosa, Staphylococcus aureus* (coagulase positive) .

EATON AGENT IDENTIFICATION

SYNONYMS:

Mycoplasma pneumoniae Identification; *M. pneumoniae* Identification.

NURSES' RESPONSIBILITY:

Any medication which the patient has been receiving must be noted on the laboratory slip. *All clinical specimens must be handled with aseptic technique.*

PRINCIPLE OF THE TEST:

M. pneumoniae (Eaton agent), a pleuropneumonia-like organism (PPLO), has been identified by a number of laboratory tests, such as indirect hemagglutination, fluorescent antibody, agglutination (plate and tube), complement-fixation, inhibition of growth (tetrazolium reduction), hemolysin production (beta-hemolytic plaque test), electrophoretic and chromatographic fractionation, culture, and paper-disc serosensitivity. Recently, a simple color test of 2, 3, 5-triphenyltetrazolium chloride (TTC) and methylene blue has been used in the diagnosis of *M. pneumoniae*. This test is based upon the inhibitory properties of various *Mycoplasma* strains by various concentrations of methylene blue chloride in agar.

At times, serial cold agglutinin studies and/or streptococcus MG agglutinin studies are used as diagnostic aids; however, these have been shown to be positive in only about one-half of all Eaton agent pneumonias.

An indirect hemagglutination test employing tanned erythrocytes and *M. pneumoniae* antigen has been used extensively, as well as the complement-fixation test.

SPECIMEN REQUIRED:

If serum is to be used, eight to ten ml of venous blood are aseptically drawn, placed in a sterile tube, and allowed to clot. The serum is separated from the clot by centrifugation. Paired sera samples—before the 10th day and after the 14th day—must be used. Other biological specimens may be used, with the test being performed as described above.

PRESERVATIVE: None is permitted.

LENGTH OF TIME REQUIRED TO PERFORM TEST:
Serologic Tests: 24 to 48 hours.
Virus Isolation: one to two weeks.
Fluorescent Antibody: one to four hours.

NORMAL VALUES: Negative for *M. pneumoniae* (Eaton agent).

POSITIVE IN:
Primary atypical pneumonia, few other pathological conditions, such as otitis media.

EYE CULTURE

A prep tray which includes the following should be set up:

Sterile swabs.

Sterile saline.

Sterile sponges.

Sterile corneal knife.

Sterile eye syringe and needles.

Most often, the ophthalmologist will prefer to collect the material from an eye disease himself. However, should the nurse be requested to obtain the specimen, the following procedure is recommended.

Procedure:

1. Anesthetize the eye with a sterile 4% solution of cocaine or a 1% solution of pentococaine.

2. Remove excessive exudates by washing the eye with a sterile saline solution.

3. Collect the material from the conjunctiva, cornea, or some other diseased part by means of a sterile swab. Return the swab to the sterile tube from which it was taken. In the case of a stye, pus should be expressed by first cleansing the surface and then expressing the pus.

4. Transport the specimen to the laboratory *immediately;* delay may result in an unsatisfactory bacteriological examination, since certain pathogens are very fragile, need moisture, and tend to die under adverse conditions. Enucleated eyes may be placed in a sterile saline solution in order to remove surface organisms.

PRINCIPLE OF THE TEST:

Material from the eye is cultured in an attempt to isolate any pathogenic organisms which may be present. The swab containing the material is rubbed onto the differential plate media (see *Culture, Routine,* p. 36), and the clock-streak method of isolation used. Cultures are usually made both aerobically and anaerobically. The differential media most often used in the isolation of pathogens from an eye are blood agar, eosin methylene blue, chocolate agar, MacConkey media, thioglycollate medium, and brain-heart infusion agar. The material may also be cultured for fungal growth (see *Fungus Culture*, p. 129) and for viral growth (see *Virus Culture*, p. 183) if the physician deems it necessary.

SPECIMEN REQUIRED: See *Nurses' Responsibility.*

PRESERVATIVE: None is permitted.

LENGTH OF TIME REQUIRED TO PERFORM TEST:

A minimum of 24 to 48 hours should be allowed for completion of a routine culture. Special cultures will require a longer period of time, depending on the specific organisms.

NORMAL VALUES: No pathogens isolated.

ABNORMAL FINDINGS:

Pathogens frequently isolated from diseases of the eye include alpha and beta streptococci, *Corynebacterium diphtheriae, Diplococcus pneumoniae, Hemophilus conjunctividitis, H. influenzae, H. parainfluenzae, Klebsiella pneumoniae, Moraxella lacunata, Neisseria gonorrhoeae, Pasteurella tularensis, Proteus vulgaris, Pseudomonas aeruginosa, Staphylococcus aureus* (coagulase positive), various viruses and fungi.

FECES, 24 - HOUR COLLECTION

Certain tests require a 24-hour collection of feces, since some substances are not uniformly excreted.

The accuracy of the 24-hour fecal collection is extremely important. Various tests require different instructions for the collection; these are listed under the *Nurses' Responsibility* heading of the respective test.

The reader is referred to the individual test for specific directions for the 24-hour fecal collection.

FECES EXAMINATION (COMPLETE)

SYNONYM: Stool Examination (Complete).

NURSES' RESPONSIBILITY:

An early morning specimen is best for a complete examination. The specimen must be fresh and contain no preservative. If it is to be mailed to a reference laboratory, the preservatives discussed below may be used. An ova and parasite examination cannot be done if barium is present.

Contamination with urine or dusting powder must be avoided. The specimen should be collected in a sterile container —preferably a bed pan—and transferred to a waxed cardboard or similar container with a tight-fitting top. A glass jar with a tight cover should *never* be used because of the buildup of gases which may cause an explosion.

The specimen may be obtained from infants from the diaper by using a sterile cotton-tipped swab. It is important that the stool specimen be kept warm if an examination for ova and parasites is to be performed.

It is often the responsibility of the nurse to observe and record the color, appearance, and quantity of the specimen.

PRINCIPLE OF THE TEST:

Normal feces consist primarily of water, food remnants, large numbers of nonpathogenic bacteria (living and dead), and undigested food remnants. A plurality of tests compose the complete fecal examination and include macroscopic, microscopic, and chemical examinations.

1. *Macroscopic Examination:* The macroscopic examination consists primarily of a description of the color and appearance of the sample, as well as careful examination for foreign bodies, such as needles, pins, and coins, that may have passed through the gastrointestinal tract.

Color: The color should be accurately described since different diseases and diets may impart various colors to the specimen.

Appearance: Normally, a rather wide range may occur in appearance of the fecal sample. The specimen may be described as hard, well formed, semisolid, or liquid. The presence of a large amount of mucus should be noted.

2. *Chemical Examination:* The chemical examination of a routine fecal examination most often consists of tests for blood and trypsin. Other tests are frequently employed.

Blood: The benzidine and guaiac tests are most frequently employed in testing the stool for occult blood. Commercial sticks and tablets based on these technics are also available for testing for blood.

Trypsin: The x-ray film method or semi-quantitative method may be used for determining tryptic activity in the stool.

3. *Microscopic Examination:* The microscopic examination most frequently includes examination of an unstained slide for pus cells, red blood cells, undigested meat fibers, vegetable fibers, bacteria, epithelial cells, and other structures which may be found in the unstained smear. Ova and parasites may be found on routine examination but frequently require special techniques. Stained slides for fat or starch may be employed.

Fat: A drop of emulsified feces is mixed with a drop of glacial acetic acid and a drop of Sudan III or Sudan IV, and the mixture is examined microscopically. Orange-red droplets indicate neutral fat. Fatty acids appear as unstained fine needles, and soaps appear as coarse, unstained crystals or irregular anthochromic globs. Upon heating, neutral fats and soaps are converted to fatty acids, which appear as large red drops. These crystallize after cooling.

Starch: Under certain conditions, such as excessive intake of raw vegetables, starch granules may appear in the feces. A small quantity of fecal material is placed on a chemically clean slide by means of an applicator stick and a drop of Lugol's solution added to stain the starch granules. The preparation is coverslipped and examined microscopically. The characteristic starch cells appear as blue-black, concentric structures. Slightly digested starch may stain red.

Ova and Parasites: Refer to page 220.

SPECIMEN REQUIRED:

A small quantity of a fresh specimen, preferably a morning specimen, is needed.

PRESERVATIVE:

Although a preservative is usually not required, the preservatives that may be used if the specimen is to be mailed to a reference laboratory for identification of ova and parasites are polyvinyl alcohol (PVA), buffered glycerol:saline, and formalin.

LENGTH OF TIME REQUIRED TO PERFORM TEST:

A minimum of one hour should be allowed for the complete examination.

NORMAL VALUES:

1. *Macroscopic Examination:*

Color: The color of normal feces depends on the amount of stercobilin (urobilin) present. Various drugs and diet may impart characteristic colors to the stool. Normally, the stool is light yellow to brown to blue-black, depending on diet, exposure to air, and the amount of urobilin present.

A *greenish-black* color may be due to ingestion of berries, iron, meat, or bismuth-containing drugs, as well as to exposure to air; *gray,* chocolate or cocoa; *yellow,* starchy foods and milk; *green,* chlorophyll from green leafy vegetables; *red,* beets; *"clay-colored",* fatty foods; *white,* ingestion of barium.

Appearance: The stool should be well formed but not hard. Mucus is usually present only in small quantities and may be seen macroscopically. The patient's diet and bowel habits may greatly influence the appearance of the specimen. For example, diets largely comprised of vegetables may result in large, soft, and predominately nonformed stools. Diets rich in protein and carbohydrates produce small, firmly formed stools. In patients suffering with constipation, the stools are frequently firm or hard, oval, or ball-shaped.

2. *Chemical Examination:* benzidine and guaiac—negative.

Blood: Negative.

Trypsin: A clear zone on the film, indicating tryptic activity; if semiquantitative tests are employed, moderate to complete digestion at the 1:10 dilution.

3. *Microscopic Examination:*

Pus cells: Few per high power field.

Red blood cells: None.

Meat fibers: Occasional one, well digested.

Vegetable fibers: Few, well digested.

Bacteria: Moderate to many, nonpathogenic.

Epithelial cells: Few per high-power field.

Ova and parasites: None found.

Fat: Negative.

Starch: Trace.

ABNORMAL FINDINGS:

1. *Macroscopic Examination:*

Color: Red streaks, usually blood from lesions in rectum or lower colon; *yellow,* fat or unchanged bilirubin; *green,* unchanged biliverdin; *gray-tan,* absence of bilirubin (due to obstructive jaundice) or excess fat due to pancreatic diseases; *black* (tarry), hemorrhage high in the gastrointestinal tract.

Appearance: Hard, grooved, or *"sheep-droppings"* appearance may be due to constipation or spastic colitis; *liquid* or *soft* and *mushy* stools, diarrhea caused by cholera, typhoid, etc., or by administration of cathartics; *flattened, ribbon-like* stools are usually found in conditions such as tumors or strictures of the rectum; *"rice-water"* stools are often seen in cases of cholera.

Normally, the amount of mucus found in the stool is extremely minute. However, in certain conditions, such as ulcerative colitis, amebiasis, intussusception, and infectious dysenteries, the quantity may be abnormally large. Large quantities of mucus signify an inflammation.

2. *Chemical Examination:*

Blood: Trace to 4^+.

Trypsin (tryptic activity): Negative.

3. *Microscopic Examination:*

Pus cells: Increased in inflammatory lesions, amebic dysentery, bacillary dysentery, bacterial diarrhea, neoplasms, syphilitic ulcers, tuberculous lesions, typhoid, ulcerative colitis.

Eosinophils: Increased in parasitic infestations, allergic conditions, neoplastic lesions of the lower intestinal tract.

Red Blood Cells: May indicate a lesion in the colon, rectum, or anus, or the presence of amoeba.

Epithelial Cells: An increase may indicate inflammation of the bowel.

Undigested Meat Fibers: An increased number of well-preserved meat fibers is found in small-intestine dysfunction due to increased peristalsis or lack of digestive juices, such as found in pancreatic insufficiency; also found in diarrhea.

Vegetable Fibers: These are important primarily because of their resemblance to the larvae of some parasites.

Bacteria: Pathogenic bacteria cannot be identified by microscopic examination of an uncultured stool. Refer to page 50 for the significance of bacterial cultures.

Crystals: The most common kind of crystals found in the feces are the *triple phosphate (ammonium magnesium phosphate); trimagnesium phosphate* crystals are found in stools exhibiting ammoniacal decomposition. A large number of *calcium oxalate* crystals are found in the stools of persons on small quantity vegetable diets; they indicate intestinal catarrh. *Charcot-Leyden* crystals may be found in parasitic infestations and in intestinal lesions of amebiasis. *Hematoidin* crystals occur after intestinal hemorrhage.

Fat: Fatty stools are frequently seen in breast-fed infants, starving people, disturbances of the biliary tract, disturbances of the mesenteric lymph nodes.

Starch: Pancreatic deficiency, excessive intake of raw vegetables, increased peristalsis in conjunction with pancreatic deficiency.

FECES (ROUTINE CULTURE FOR BACTERIA)

SYNONYM: Stool Culture (Routine).

NURSES' RESPONSIBILITY:

The stool specimen must be collected in a sterile container, avoiding contamination with urine or dusting powder. Disposable receptables are preferred. If it is necessary to transfer a portion from a sterile bedpan to a smaller receptacle, a sterile spatula must be used. The specimen should be refrigerated if it cannot be cultured immediately, since nonpathogenic organisms tend to overgrow and obscure many of the pathogenic organisms that may be present.

Since only a very small specimen is needed for culture of the organisms, a sterile swab may be inserted into the rectum and the specimen obtained. Swabs should be placed directly into a tube of enrichment broth to assure viability of the organisms.

If the patient has chronic dysentery, it is preferable to obtain material by means of a rectal swab during proctoscopic examination. The material should be cultured immediately since *Shigella* and certain other organisms have a short survival time.

PRINCIPLE OF THE TEST:

Pathogenic bacteria may be isolated and differentiated from nonpathogenic bacteria by culturing on selective media. Selective media for the isolation of enteric bacteria most often include Hektoen enteric, blood agar, eosinmethylene blue (EMB), Endo agar, Salmonella-Shigella (SS) agar/MacConkey agar, and Staph 110 medium.

A small quantity of the specimen is inoculated onto the media by means of a platinum inoculating loop. The organisms are also cultured in an enrichment broth. At the end of 24 hours incubation, the plates and broth tubes are examined for particular characteristic growth or organisms. A Gram stain (see p. 59) is usually a part of the complete culture examination, with subsequent microscopic examination.

SPECIMEN REQUIRED:

A small quantity of fecal specimen, collected by sterile technique, is needed.

PRESERVATIVE:

None is permitted, since it may inhibit the growth of organisms.

LENGTH OF TIME REQUIRED TO PERFORM TEST:

A minimum of 24 to 48 hours should be allowed.

NORMAL FINDINGS:

Organisms considered as nonpathogens are *Alcaligenes fecalis, Bacteroides, Escherichia coli, Lactobacillus acidophilus;* various yeast forms, including *Candida albicans,* may be present normally, but mycelial filaments of *C. albicans* are considered pathogenic.

VARIABLE PATHOGENICITY:

The following *may* be pathogenic when found in fecal specimens: *Aerobacter aerogenes, Clostridium perfringens, Escherichia freundii, Klebsiella pneumoniae, Mycobacterium tuberculosis, Proteus* spp., *Serratia marcescens,* others.

PATHOGENIC FINDINGS:

The following organisms are considered pathogenic when found in the feces: *Proteus* (certain species) , *Pseudomonas aeruginosa, Salmonella paratyphi, S. typhosa, Shigella* spp., *Staphylococcus aureus* (coagulase positive) , *Vibrio comma, Candida albicans* (mycelial filaments) .

FLUORESCENT ANTIBODY TEST

SYNONYMS: FA Test, Immunofluorescence Technique.

NURSES' RESPONSIBILITY:

No special preparation of the patient is needed.

PRINCIPLE OF THE TEST:

The fluorescent antibody test is employed as a means of detecting antigen-antibody reactions. The material to be examined, containing the antigen, is labeled with a fluorescent-tagged antibody solution such as fluorescein, nuclear-fast red, rhodamine B, or auramine. The antigen-antibody conjugation fluoresces upon irradiation with ultraviolet light under a fluorescent microscope.

The test is a specific staining procedure. Controls are always performed in conjunction with the actual test procedure. Chief advantage of the test is the rapidity with which it may be performed.

Four methods of FA staining are currently being utilized.

1. *Direct:* This is the simplest procedure. The material containing the antigen (source of the antigen) is placed on a glass slide containing special wells and designed for fluorescence microscopy work. The source of antigen may consist of serum, tissue culture, frozen sections, impression smears, or throat washings which have been fixed to the slide by methanol, acetone, heat, or other means. The known *labeled* antiserum is applied to the test material at 37°C for approximately 15 minutes. This time may vary, depending on the system under study. After the 15-minute period, the excess unreacted fluorescent material is washed away by means of phosphate-buffered saline, the preparation mounted in buffered glycerol, and the slide examined by a fluorescence microscope.

2. *Inhibition:* The material containing the antigen (source of antigen) is placed on a glass slide with special wells designed for fluorescence microscopy work. The test material is exposed to a specific *unlabeled* antibody at 37°C for approximately 15 minutes, the excess unreacted fluorescent material washed away, and the preparation mounted and examined under the fluorescence microscope.

This procedure "blocks" the usual antigen-antibody reaction; therefore, there is no fluorescence but rather inhibition.

3. *Indirect:* The material containing the unlabeled antigen (source of antigen) is placed on a glass slide containing wells and designed for fluorescence microscopy work. *Unlabeled* antiserum is applied to the preparation for 15 to 30 minutes and the excess material washed away. Fluorescence indicates an unlabeled product. The preparation is then allowed to react with a *labeled* antiglobulin for determination of the labeled product, and is washed, mounted, and examined in the usual manner.

4. *Complement Staining:* This procedure is very similar to that employed for the indirect method. The test material (source of antigen) is placed on a glass slide containing special wells designed for fluorescence microscopy work. A fixed quantity of guinea pig complement and inactivated primary reagent serum are added simultaneously to the antigen. This conjugate is washed and incubated at 37°C for approximately 15 minutes. A second step is employed in which anti-guinea pig complement is added and the preparation reincubated. The slide is washed, mounted, and examined in the usual manner.

Currently, fluorescent antibody studies are being used in many fields, such as diagnostic parasitology, bacteriology, virology, rickettsiology, immunology, and numerous others.

Since the rabies virus is considered to be one of the most highly neurotropic viruses, as well as one of extreme importance, a separate procedure has been described under *Rabies Virus,* page 174.

The following procedure is frequently used in preparing the material for the staining process.

Procedure:

1. Place a small quantity of the test material in the well of a slide designed for fluorescent antibody work.

2. Immerse the slide in a Coplin jar containing acetone or some other fixing agent.

3. Refrigerate and allow to "fix" as −20°C for four hours.

4. Stain by one of the four methods previously described.

SPECIMEN REQUIRED:

Serum, plasma, whole blood, throat washings, tissue culture, feces, exudates, or any material in which the fluorescent antibody technique might be of value.

LENGTH OF TIME REQUIRED TO PERFORM TEST:

A minimum of one to two hours must be allowed.

NORMAL VALUES: No fluorescence of pathological organisms.

POSITIVE FINDINGS IN:

The following organisms have been identified by the fluorescent antibody method: Arbor viruses (group B), *Bacillus anthracis, Blastomyces dermatiditis* (yeast form), *Bordetella pertussis, Brucella* spp., *Clostridium* spp., *Coccidioides immitis, Corynebacterium diphtheriae, Cryptococcus neoformans, Endamoeba coli, E. histolytica, Erysipelothrix insidiosa, Escherichia coli,* herpes simplex virus, *Histoplasma capsulatum,* influenza virus, *Leptospira* spp., *Listeria monocytogenes,* lymphocytic choriomeningitis virus, *Mycobacterium tuberculosis, Mycoplasma pneumoniae* (Eaton Agent), *Pasteurella* spp., poliomyelitis virus, *Pseudomonas* spp., psittacosis virus, rabies virus, *Salmonella* spp., Sendai virus, *Shigella* spp., *Staphylococcus* spp., *Streptococcus* spp., *Toxoplasma gondii, Treponema pallidum,* vaccinia virus, *Vibrio fetus,* many others.

GASTRIC WASHINGS FOR TUBERCLE BACILLI

SYNONYMS:

Gastric Washings for Acid-fast Bacilli, Gastric Washings for *Mycobacterium tuberculosis.*

NURSES' RESPONSIBILITY:

The patient should be instructed to fast for 12 hours prior to the start of this test, to prevent obstruction of the tube by food particles.

It should be stressed at this time that care must be taken to avoid contamination of both personnel and room. It should be remembered that *all gastric washings for tubercle bacilli must be considered to be positive until they are proven to be negative.* Strict *isolation* technique must be employed from the beginning of the procedure. All personnel must wear caps, masks, and gowns. The working area must be covered with disposable sheets or towels, or those that may be sterilized immediately following the procedure. Disposable gloves should be used also.

The fasting contents are aspirated with a disposable plastic tube and a 50 ml syringe; they are placed in a sterile conical culture tube with cap, labeled *fasting specimen.* Sterile 0.85% saline is warmed to 37°C and 30 ml of the normal saline is injected with a sterile syringe through the gastric tube into the stomach. This is aspirated with the syringe and placed into another container with cap, marked *first washing.* This procedure is repeated three or four times, using a different sterile culture tube for each washing. Each tube must be carefully labeled. All washings must be sent to the laboratory *immediately* for testing.

Extreme caution should be taken to incinerate all disposable materials immediately, and the nonexpendables must be sterilized. A disinfectant should be applied to any part of the room which has been accidentally contaminated.

PRINCIPLE OF THE TEST:

Patients who are infected with the tubercle bacillus *(Mycobacterium tuberculosis)* frequently cough up and swallow the organism. Gastric contents, when cultured, often yield growth of the organism from infected patients. Refer to *Tuberculosis Study (Sputum)*, page 99.

SPECIMEN REQUIRED:

A few milliliters of freshly aspirated gastric washings are needed.

PRESERVATIVE:

None is permitted. The contents should be placed in a clean, sterile container. Any preservative may kill the organism, causing false results.

LENGTH OF TIME REQUIRED TO PERFORM TEST:

One hour should be allowed for the aspiration. The cultures are examined daily for growth. The negative culture must be incubated for six to eight weeks before it can be reported.

NORMAL VALUES:

Negative culture: No organisms characteristic of *Mycobacterium tuberculosis* isolated.

Direct smear: No acid-fast bacilli characteristic of *Mycobacterium tuberculosis* seen.

POSITIVE IN: Tuberculosis.

GELATIN LIQUEFACTION BY BACTERIA

SYNONYM: Bacterial Liquefaction of Gelatin.

NURSES' RESPONSIBILITY:

No special preparation of the patient is needed.

PRINCIPLE OF THE TEST:

Certain bacterial organisms have the ability to liquefy a gelatin medium. A gelatin medium is stabbed with a wire inoculating loop with the test organisms on it, and the medium is incubated at 20-22°C. After the incubation period, the tube is refrigerated at 4-6°C for 30 minutes and the test recorded as:

Positive: No solidification of gelatin.

Negative: Solidification of gelatin.

An alternate method includes streaking a plate of nutrient agar with the test organism, incubating it at 28°C for two to four days, and covering it with a mercuric chloride solution. The test is reported as follows:

Positive (liquefaction): Clear zone of changed gelatin.

Negative (no liquefaction): White opaque precipitate but unchanged gelatin.

SPECIMEN REQUIRED: A few colonies of the test organism are needed.

PRESERVATIVE: None is permitted.

LENGTH OF TIME REQUIRED TO PERFORM TEST:

A minimum of 24 hours from the time of inoculation of the gelatin is needed; it may take as long as four days before a final report is made.

POSITIVE IN:

Aerobacter aerogenes, Arizona, Bacillus anthracis, Chromobacterium spp., *Clostridium* spp. (some), *Erysipelothrix insidiosa, Flavobacterium meningosepticum, Proteus* spp. (some), *Pseudomonas aeruginosa, Nocardia asteroides, Serratia marcescens, Streptococcus* spp.

NEGATIVE IN:

Actinomyces spp., *Brucella* spp., *Clostridium* spp. (some), *Corynebacterium acnes, Escherichia coli, E. freundii, Hafnia* spp.,

Klebsiella pneumoniae, Listeria monocytogenes, Lactobacillus bifidus, Nocardia spp. (some) , *Proteus* spp. (some) , *Providencia* spp., *Salmonella* spp., *Shigella* spp., *Streptococcus* spp. (some), few others.

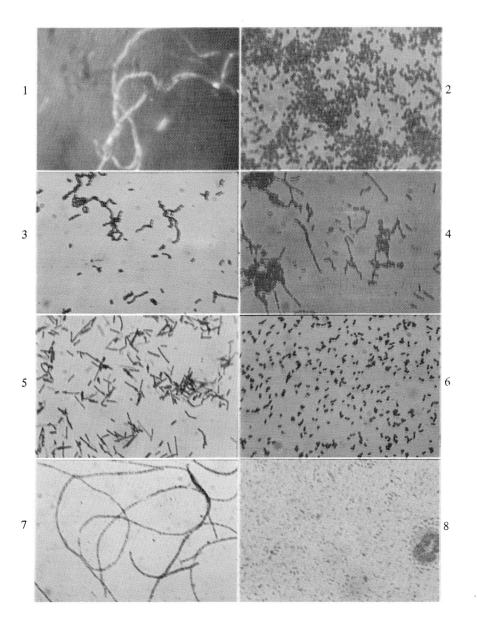

1. *Bacillus anthracis* organisms stained by fluoroscein isothiocyanate for fluorescent antibody determination.
3. *Streptococcus pyogenes.*
5. *Corynebacterium pyogenes.*
7. *Bacillus anthracis.*

2. *Staphylococcus aureus.*
4. *Erysipelothrix insidiosa.*
6. *Listeria monocytogenes.*
8. *Diplococcus pneumoniae.*

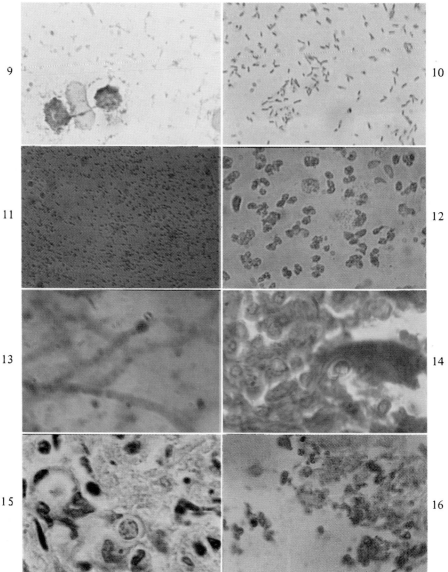

9. *Hemophilus influenzae.*

10. *Escherichia coli.*

11. *Brucella abortus.*

12. *Neisseria gonorrhoeae:* Gonococci from a cervical smear showing pus cells and typical gram-negative intracellular coccobacilli.

13. *Aspergillus fumigatus:* From a patient with otomycosis.

14. *Blastomyces dermatitidis.*

15. *Blastomyces dermatitidis:* Smear showing double-contoured ring with chromatin in center.

16. *Cryptococcus neoformans:* Smear showing cryptococci; found in spinal fluid.

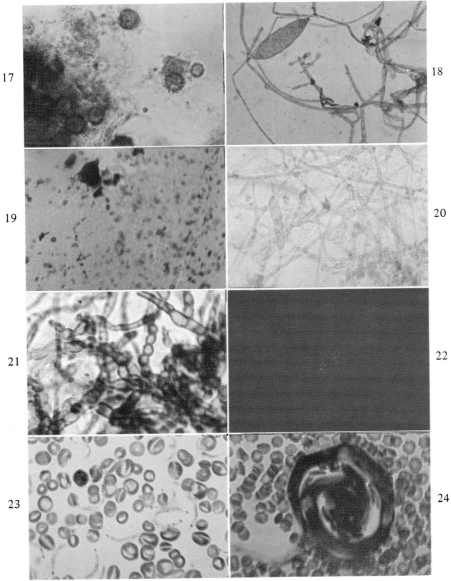

17. *Histoplasma capsulatum:* Smear from rectal ulcer showing oval, intracellular, yeastlike fungi.

19. *Sporotrichum schenckii:* Smear showing clusters of spores from an inoculated mouse.

21. *Phialaphora verrucosa:* Culture showing dark brown to olive-green irregular cells.

23. *Trypanosoma lewisi:* From blood of infected rat.

18. *Microsporum gypseum:* Smear from scalp; fuseaux are blunt and club-shaped.

20. *Hormodendrum pedrosoi:* Culture showing multiple, branch-like chains.

22. Negri body, stained by fluorescent antibody.

24. Filarial larvae in blood.

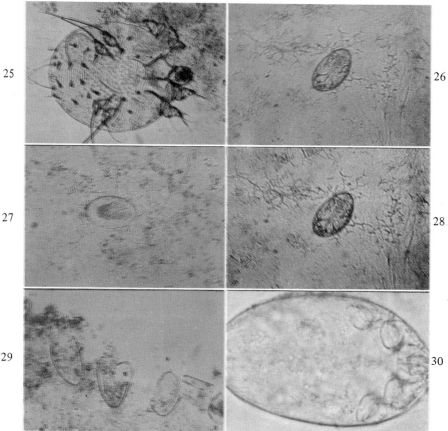

25. *Sarcoptes scabiei:* Mature form.
26. *S. scabiei:* Form ready to hatch.
27. *S. scabiei:* Infertile ovum.
28. *S. scabiei:* Ovum.
29. *S. scabiei:* Empty ovum.
30. *S. scabiei:* Immature — in ovum.

GRAM STAIN (HUCKER MODIFICATION)

NURSES' RESPONSIBILITY:

No special preparation of the patient is needed.

PRINCIPLE OF THE TEST:

When stained with a crystal violet solution, all organisms absorb the dye. However, upon the addition of Gram's iodine solution, which acts as a mordant, certain organisms retain the dye when treated with an alcohol-acetone decolorizing agent while others do not. This procedure divides the bacteria into two groups. The organisms which retain the dye are known as *gram-positive* organisms; those not retaining the dye are known as *gram-negative* organisms. The gram-negative organisms stain red with a counterstain such as safranin or dilute carbolfuchsin, while the gram-positive organisms do not pick up the counterstain and so remain blue.

The Gram stain is an extremely important diagnostic aid in bacteriological studies. The procedure is relatively simple.

Procedure:

1. Flood the fixed slide with crystal violet stain and allow to stain for 30 to 60 seconds.

2. Pour off the stain by tipping the slide.

3. Flood with iodine solution to allow to mordant for one minute.

4. Rinse with tap water.

5. Decolorize with alcohol-acetone solution until the solvent appears colorless. This is approximately 30 seconds.

6. Counterstain with safranin or some similar counterstain for approximately 30 seconds.

7. Wash with tap water, blot dry, and examine under oil immersion.

SPECIMEN REQUIRED:

This may be either a direct smear obtained from the immediate source, or a smear prepared from an 18 to 24 hour culture of organisms.

PRESERVATIVE: None is required.

LENGTH OF TIME REQUIRED TO PERFORM TEST:

A minimum of 30 minutes should be allowed.

GRAM-POSITIVE:

Representatives of bacteria stained by Gram's stain include the following:

1. Bacilli:

    Bacillus anthracis, B. subtilis, Clostridium tetani, Corynebacterium diphtheriae, C. hofmanni, C. xerosis, Erysipelothrix insidiosa, Lactobacillus acidophilus, Listeria monocytogenes, Mycobacterium leprae, M. smegmatis, M. tuberculosis.

2. Cocci:

    Diplococcus pneumoniae, Gaffkya tetragena, Sarcina lutea, Staphylococcus aureus, S. epidermidis, Streptococcus pyogenes, S. viridans.

GRAM-NEGATIVE:

1. Bacilli:

    Aerobacter aerogenes, Bacteroides fragilis, Bacillus fusiformis, Bordetella pertussis, Borrelia vincentii, Brucella abortus, B. suis, B. melitensis, Escherichia coli, Hemophilus ducreyi, H. influenzae, Klebsiella pneumoniae, Moraxella lacunata, Pasteurella multocida, Pasteurella pestis, Pasteurella tularensis, Proteus vulgaris, Pseudomonas aeruginosa, Salmonella typhosa, Shigella sonnei, Vibrio comma, Vibrio fetus.

2. Cocci:

    Neisseria catarrhalis, N. gonorrhoeae, N. haemolysans, N. meningitidis, N. sicca.

HYDROGEN SULFIDE TEST

SYNONYM: H₂S Test for Bacterial Identification.

NURSES' RESPONSIBILITY:

No special preparation of the patient is needed.

PRINCIPLE OF THE TEST:

Certain organisms have the ability to produce hydrogen sulfide when inoculated into a medium such as basic lead acetate broth.

A few colonies of the test organisms are placed in a peptone-agar basic lead acetate solution, and the color reaction is observed. Hydrogen sulfide is produced from the sulfur-containing amino acids of the medium. This is observed as a brownish-black color of the compound, lead sulfide, which has been formed by the combination of hydrogen sulfide with lead acetate. The test is reported as follows:

Black or brown color: Positive.

No change in color: Negative.

Other selective media which are of benefit in determining hydrogen sulfide production include triple sugar medium (TSI), bismuth citrate, ferrous sulfate, ferric citrate, or lead acetate paper.

SPECIMEN REQUIRED: A few colonies of the test organism are needed.

PRESERVATIVE: None is permitted.

LENGTH OF TIME REQUIRED TO PERFORM TEST:

A minimum of seven days should be allowed for reporting of negative reactions.

NORMAL VALUES:

There are no set normal values for this test.

POSITIVE IN:

Bacteroides fragilis, Brucella spp., *Clostridium* spp. (some), *Escherichia freundii, Flavobacterium meningosepticum, Hafnia* sp., *Listeria monocytogenes, Pasteurella multocida, Proteus* spp. *(some), Pa. pseudotuberculosis, Salmonella* spp., *Serratia marcescens.*

NEGATIVE IN: Most others not mentioned above.

IMViC REACTIONS

This mnemonic formula (IMViC) refers to the four biochemical tests used in the identification of the coliform bacilli: *indole, methyl red, Voges-Proskauer,* and *citrate utilization.* There are 16 possible combinations of positive and negative tests of these four characteristics.

The reader is referred to the individual tests which are listed alphabetically in this book as follows:

Indole (I), page 63.
Methyl Red (M), page 65.
Voges-Proskauer (Vi), page 107.
Citrate Utilization (C), page 33.

INDOLE TEST

SYNONYMS:
Oxalic Acid Paper Test, Kovac's Indole Test, Gnezda's Test for Indole.

NURSES' RESPONSIBILITY:
No special preparation of the patient is needed.

PRINCIPLE OF THE TEST:
Certain bacteria have the ability to produce indole from tryptophane. A tryptone broth solution is inoculated with a few test colonies, and the mixture is incubated at 37°C for 48 hours. A few drops of Kovac's reagent (paradimethylaminobenzaldehyde solution) are added and the color reaction observed as follows:

Cherry red: Positive.

Colorless: Negative.

An alternate method is the oxalic acid paper (Gnezda) test. This employs a strip of filter paper impregnated with a saturated solution of oxalic acid. When the strip is inserted into the incubated culture, a pink color indicates an indole production. No change in the strip indicates a negative test.

SPECIMEN REQUIRED: A few colonies of the test organism are needed.

PRESERVATIVE: None is required.

LENGTH OF TIME REQUIRED TO PERFORM TEST:
A minimum of 48 hours including growth of the test organism is needed.

POSITIVE IN:
Clostridium spp. (some), *Escherichia coli, Flavobacterium meningosepticum, Proteus morganii, P. rettgeri, P. vulgaris, Providencia* spp., *Shigella* spp., *Vibrio comma.*

NEGATIVE IN:
Aerobacter aerogenes, Alcaligenes fecalis, Clostridium spp. (some), *Escherichia coli, Klebsiella pneumoniae, Pseudomonas* spp., *Salmonella* spp., *Proteus mirabilis, Serratia marcescens, Shigella sonnei.*

MEMBRANE FILTER TECHNIQUE

SYNONYM: Millipore Membrane Filter Technique.

NURSES' RESPONSIBILITY:

No special preparation of the patient is needed.

PRINCIPLE OF THE TEST:

When fluids are passed through a thin plastic and porous filter known as a membrane filter, all particles larger than the pores of the filter are retained on the surface of the filter.

The membrane filter is composed of pure inert cellulose esters; they are found in various pore sizes (ranging from 5 microns to 10 millimicrons), and they exhibit an extremely uniform size of pores. The filter is most often attached to a special holder for convenience of operation.

The material retained on the surface of the filter is processed in the same way as for a bacterial or fungus culture for identification, or a cytology smear. The membrane filter technique has proven itself in the past and is continuing to be widely used in the identification of particulate matter, bacteria, and cells present in gases and liquids.

SPECIMEN REQUIRED:

Any particulate matter, bacteria, or cells may be processed.

PRESERVATIVE: None is required.

LENGTH OF TIME REQUIRED TO PERFORM TEST:

This will depend on the type of material being filtered, and also on the tests performed following the filtration.

NORMAL VALUES: There are no set normal values for this test.

ABNORMAL FINDINGS:

Any pathogenic organisms or cells which may be isolated by other techniques may be identified through the use of this procedure.

METHYL RED TEST

SYNONYM: M.R. Test for Bacteria.

NURSES' RESPONSIBILITY:

No special preparation of the patient is needed.

PRINCIPLE OF THE TEST:

Certain organisms have the ability to produce a high acidity from dextrose in a glucose phosphate broth, and they therefore cause a color reaction to occur when an alcoholic methyl red indicator solution is added. The test is reported as follows:

Red color (distinct): Positive.

Yellow color: Negative.

The test is most often employed in the differentiation of *Aerobacter* and *Escherichia.*

SPECIMEN REQUIRED: A few colonies of the test organism are needed.

PRESERVATIVE: None is required.

LENGTH OF TIME REQUIRED TO PERFORM TEST:

A minimum of two to three days should be allowed.

POSITIVE IN:

Escherichia coli, Escherichia freundii, Hafnia, Listeria monocytogenes, Pasteurella pseudotuberculosis, Proteus spp., *Providencia* spp., *Salmonella* spp., *Shigella* spp., few others.

NEGATIVE IN:

Aerobacter aerogenes, most other organisms not mentioned above.

MOTILITY TESTS FOR BACTERIA

Nurses' Responsibility:

No special preparation of the patient is needed.

Principle of the Test:

Bacteria that possess flagella are considered to be motile. Motility may be demonstrated by microscopic hanging-drop preparations or inoculation into a semisolid medium.

Semisolid Medium: Certain bacteria exhibit the ability to remain motile when inoculated onto a select semisolid medium ("motility medium"). The organisms are stabbed onto the top of the column of medium to a depth of 5 to 10 mm, and the test is observed at 8, 24, and 48 hours. The test is reported as follows:

Positive (motile): Growth throughout the medium.

Negative (nonmotile): Growth along the stab line only.

Hanging-Drop Preparation: An alternate method is the hanging-drop preparation. This is most frequently used for the determination of motility of young cultures (18 hours or less). A few colonies of the test organism are suspended in a drop of saline or broth on a coverglass which is inverted on a "well" slide. The preparation is then viewed for motility of the organisms by phase-contrast microscopy or by visible light microscopy using a reduced light. True motility must not be confused with Brownian movement (movement caused by bombardment of the molecules).

Specimen Required: A few colonies of the test organism are needed.

Preservative: None is permitted.

Length of Time Required to Perform Test:

A minimum of four hours should be allowed.

Normal Values:

There is no correlation between motility and pathogenicity.

Positive in:

Some of the organisms in which the test is positive include. *Aerobacter aerogenes, Alcaligenes fecalis, Clostridium* spp. (most), *Escherichia coli, Proteus vulgaris, Pseudomonas aeruginosa, Salmonella typhosa, Spirillum volutans,* others.

NEISSERIA GONORRHOEAE (IDENTIFICATION)

SYNONYMS: *N. gonorrhoeae* Test, Gonococcus Test, G.C. Test.

NURSES' RESPONSIBILITY:

A prep tray containing the following materials should be set up:

Sterile inoculating loops.
Chemically clean glass slides.
Sterile cotton-tipped swabs.
Sterile containers for prostatic fluid or urine.

The exudate from the vaginal secretions of the female, or the urethra of the male, should be collected on a sterile inoculating loop, smeared on a chemically clean glass slide, and air-dried. The slide *must* be brought to the laboratory immediately for identification by Gram staining. If the disease in males has migrated into the urinary tract, it may be necessary for the physician to perform a prostatic massage. In such a case, the specimen must be collected in a sterile container and brought to the laboratory immediately without delay.

The urine or other suspected material may also be cultured for *N. gonorrhoeae*. The specimen must be collected in a sterile container and transported to the laboratory for immediate culturing. If the specimen cannot be cultured for several hours, the material should be collected on cotton swabs, immersed in a mixture of broth, gentian violet, starch, and holding broth.

PRINCIPLE OF THE TEST:

In some diseases such as acute urethritis in males, and vaginitis in females, the infective agent is *N. gonorrhoeae* (gonococcus). This is a gram-negative, bean-shaped diplococcus that occurs within polymorphonuclear leukocytes on a Gram-stained slide. A few of the organisms may be found extracellularly.

In most cases, the diagnostician may wish to culture the specimen. The medium of choice is either chocolate blood agar or GC medium, both of which require 10% carbon dioxide for producing growth of the organism. The cultures are incubated at 35°C for 24 to 48 hours. Cultural techniques have been shown to reveal almost twice as many positives as did direct smears.

The fluorescent antibody method (p. 52) of diagnosis may also be of assistance. The gonococcus has been shown to possess a specific K-type antigen, thereby enabling the identification of the organism.

Identification of the isolated organism may be further verified by the oxidase test, page 73.

SPECIMEN REQUIRED: Refer to *Nurses' Responsibility.*

PRESERVATIVE: None is permitted.

LENGTH OF TIME REQUIRED TO PERFORM TEST:

A minimum of one hour should be allowed for the smear examination, one hour for the fluorescent antibody procedure, and 24 to 48 hours for the culture.

NORMAL VALUES:

Smear: Negative (no intracellular or extracellular gram-negative diplococci characteristic of *N. gonorrhoeae* found) .

Culture: No organisms characteristic of *N. gonorrhoeae* isolated.

Fluorescent antibody: No fluoresence of *N. gonorrhoeae* organisms seen.

NITRATE REDUCTION TEST

Synonyms: Ilosvay's Test, Nitroso Reaction.

Nurses' Responsibility:
No special preparation of the patient is needed.

Principle of the Test:
Certain organisms have the ability to utilize nitrates as hydrogen receptors, reducing the nitrate (NO_3) radical to nitrite (NO_2) when in the presence of alpha-naphthylamine-acetic acid: sulfanilic acid.

A few colonies of the test organism are inoculated by stabbing into a peptone medium for aerobic organisms. For anaerobic organisms, an anaerobic nitrate broth is used. The test reaction is read in one to three minutes and reported as follows:

Pink—deep red: Positive.

Colorless: Negative.

If no color develops, one may assume the absence of nitrite and hence no reduction of nitrate, or that both the nitrite and nitrate have been reduced. Negative tests may be verified by adding a small quantity of zinc dust to the culture. Development of a red color shows evidence of unreduced nitrate.

Specimen Required:
A few colonies of the test organism are needed.

Preservative: None is required.

Length of Time Required to Perform Test:
A minimum of 30 minutes following previous growth of the test organism should be allowed.

Positive in:
Actinomyces spp., *Chromobacterium* spp., *Corynebacterium acnes, Clostridium* spp. (some), *Pasteurella multocida, Pseudomonas aeruginosa, Serratia marcescens,* few others.

Negative in: Others not listed above.

OPSONIC INDEX FOR TULAREMIA

SYNONYM: Opsonophagocytic Test for Tularemia.

NURSES' RESPONSIBILITY:

Since tularemia is a highly contagious disease with a mortality rate as high as 5% to 6%, it is essential that the utmost precautions be taken when working with the patient or his biological specimens.

The patient need not be fasting or in a resting state for this test.

PRINCIPLE OF THE TEST:

A quantitative estimate of opsonin of a specific immune serum is compared to the number of bacteria phagocytized by an arbitrary number of normal leukocytes in the specific immune serum.

The test is used primarily in the determination of immunity to tularemia and for proper diagnosis must be run in conjunction with the tularemia agglutination test and Foshay's test.

The test is based on the ability of the polymorphonuclear leukocytes to ingest or phagocytize the *Pasteurella tularensis* organism. One-tenth milliliter of the patient's citrated blood is added to a suspension of *P. tularensis* organisms (formalin-killed and formalin-free) and incubated 30 minutes at 37°C. The sedimented cells are spread on a chemically clean glass slide and stained with an aniline dye. They are then observed for phagocytosis for enumeration of the bacteria that have been ingested by an arbitrary number (usually 50) of polymorphonuclear leukocytes. The test is reported as follows:

Negative: No phagocytosis.

Slight Phagocytosis: 1 to 20 phagocytized bacteria per neutrophil.

Moderate Phagocytosis: 21-40 phagocytized bacteria per neutrophil.

Marked Phagocytosis: 41 or more phagocytized bacteria per neutrophil.

SPECIMEN REQUIRED:

Five milliliters of venous blood are withdrawn and added to 0.2 ml 20% sodium citrate in a sterile tube.

PRESERVATIVE:

None is required. The test must be performed within six hours to avoid disintegration of the leukocytes.

LENGTH OF TIME REQUIRED TO PERFORM TEST:

A minimum of two hours should be allowed.

NORMAL VALUES:

Sixty percent or more of the segmented neutrophils showing marked phagocytosis.

POSITIVE IN:

Active tularemia infections or immunity to tularemia.

OPTOCHIN DISC TEST

SYNONYM: Ethylhydrocupreine Hydrochloride Test.

NURSES' RESPONSIBILITY:

No special preparation of the patient is needed.

PRINCIPLE OF THE TEST:

This test is used primarily in the differentiation of *pneumo-cocci* spp. and *streptococci* spp.

A blood agar plate is inoculated with the suspected organism, and a small sterile paper disc impregnated with optochin (ethyl-hydrocupreine hydrochloride) is placed on the plate. If the pneumococcus organism is present, a large zone (15 to 30 mm in diameter) of inhibition around the disc is evident, whereas *alpha-Streptococcus* organisms are not inhibited and thereby produce no zone. The test appears to be directly correlated with bile solubility.

SPECIMEN REQUIRED:

A few colonies of the test organism obtained from an overnight primary culture or a pure culture are needed.

LENGTH OF TIME REQUIRED TO PERFORM TEST:

A minimum of 24 hours should be allowed.

PRESERVATIVE: None is required.

NORMAL VALUES: There are no set normal values for this test.

GROWTH ZONE INHIBITION IN: Pneumococcus *(Diplococcus pneumoniae)*.

GROWTH UNAFFECTED IN: *alpha-Streptococcus. (Streptococcus Viridans)*

OXIDASE TEST

SYNONYMS:
Cytochrome Oxidase Test, Gaby's Oxidase Test, Ewing-Johnson Oxidase Test.

NURSES' RESPONSIBILITY:
No special preparation of the patient is needed.

PRINCIPLE OF THE TEST:
Certain bacteria, such as the *Neisseria,* contain an enzyme, known as *oxidase* which is capable of oxidation. These bacteria, when in contact with a dilute 1% dimethylparaphenylenediamine chloride or tetramethylparaphenylenediamine dihydrochloride solution, produce a colored compound which indicates the presence of cytochrome oxidase.

The organisms to be tested are incubated approximately 18 to 20 hours on nutrient agar slants or blood agar plates. A few milliliters of the test reagent are dropped onto the test colonies and the color reaction observed within 30 to 60 seconds as follows:

Pink—maroon: Positive.

Colorless: Negative.

The test may also be performed using commercial discs impregnated with the above reagents.

The oxidase test is usually run in conjunction with other studies for gonorrhea and meningitis, such as the typical fermentation of sugars. It is also used in the differentiation of *Aeromonas* and other similar groups from groups such as the *Aerobacter.*

SPECIMEN REQUIRED:
A few colonies of the test organism previously cultured on either nutrient agar or blood agar are needed.

PRESERVATIVE: None is permitted.

LENGTH OF TIME REQUIRED TO PERFORM TEST:
A minimum of 30 minutes should be allowed.

POSITIVE IN:
Groups of *Aeromonas, Alcaligenes, Neisseria, Pseudomonas, Vibrio,* others.

Negative in:

Groups of *Aerobacter, Arizona, Escherichia, Hafnia, Klebsiella, Proteus, Providencia, Salmonella, Serratia, Shigella,* others.

PHAGE TYPING

SYNONYMS:

Bacteriophage Typing, Bacteriolysin Typing, "Phage Pattern."

NURSES' RESPONSIBILITY:

No special preparation of the patient is needed.

PRINCIPLE OF THE TEST:

A viral agent known as "phage" (bacteriophage) has been shown to exhibit a lytic activity upon certain bacterial cells.

Bacteriophage typing has been of particular use in the typing and strain differentiation of certain genera of microorganisms, particularly those of the staphylococci. The typing phages all belong to the general class, "phages with restricted host range."

A blood agar plate is inoculated with a generous bacterial culture to provide confluent growth. Several drops each of a variety of phage types are placed at various positions on the surface of the agar, and the plate is incubated at 37°C for four to eighteen hours. Thereafter, the number of *plaques* that have been produced by each phage is recorded. Plaques are "pinholes" or areas in which no visible bacterial growth has occurred. The presence or absence of the phage plaques gives rise to the "phage pattern." The plaques are determined with the aid of a bright light and a dark background. Moderate magnification may be accomplished by the use of a hand lens, Quebec colony counter, or a stereoscopic microscope.

Several methods are available for reporting of the phage types. The following is one of the more frequently used:

(Weak) ±: 0 to 20 plaques.

(Moderate) +: 20 to 50 plaques.

(Strong) ++: 50 plaques to confluent lysis.

The phage type is usually reported as the number of phages giving a ++ (strong reaction). For example, if phage numbers 6, 53, 54, and 75 give a ++ reaction, the reading would be reported as ++: 6/53/54/75. The number of plaques formed is *directly* proportional to the number of phage particles in the test sample.

Another system of reporting shows the phages giving *complete* lysis first. This is followed by a slant line; those giving a ++ reaction, followed by a colon; reaction easily read, followed by a slant line; and the weak reactions are last in position. For example, the phage pattern would be reported as 6,7/47,53,54:75/77.

Since there is such a vast number of typing phages for routine work, the International Subcommittee usually recommends a basic set to be used in the particular situation.

SPECIMEN REQUIRED:

A few colonies of a six to eighteen hour bacterial culture are needed.

PRESERVATIVE: None is permitted.

LENGTH OF TIME REQUIRED TO PERFORM TEST:

A minimum of 18 to 36 hours should be allowed.

NORMAL VALUES:

Since there is no laboratory test for demonstrating the virulence for man, evaluation must be based on clinical and epidemiological findings. Refer to *principle of the test* and *significance of findings* for further discussion.

SIGNIFICANCE OF FINDINGS:

Phage typings have been useful in many diagnostic procedures, including those of staphylococcal disease, food poisonings, pemphigus neonatorum, wound infections, furunculosis, postoperative infections, and postnatal infection.

Phage typings have been performed for many different bacterial species, a few of which are *Bacillus anthracis, Corynebacterium diphtheriae, Escherichia coli, Pseudomonas aeruginosa, Salmonella* spp., *Staphylococcus* spp., *Streptococcus lactis.*

PHENYLALANINE DEAMINASE TEST FOR BACTERIAL IDENTIFICATION

NURSES' RESPONSIBILITY:

No special preparation of the patient is needed.

PRINCIPLE OF THE TEST:

Certain bacteria, such as those in Enterobacteriaceae, have the ability to form phenylpyruvic acid from phenylalanine by deamination.

A slant of phenylalanine agar is inoculated with the test organism and incubated at 37°C for 24 hours. After the incubation period, a few drops of ferric chloride are allowed to run onto the inoculum. The test is reported as follows:

Green Color (phenylpyruvic acid present): Positive.

Absence of Green Color (no phenylpyruvic acid present): Negative.

The test is used most frequently in differentiating the *Proteus–Providencia* organisms from the Enterobacteriaceae.

SPECIMEN REQUIRED: A few colonies of the test organisms are needed.

PRESERVATIVE: None is permitted.

LENGTH OF TIME REQUIRED TO PERFORM TEST:

A minimum of 12 to 24 hours following growth of the original culture must be allowed.

POSITIVE IN:

Groups of *Aerobacter, Arizona, Citrobacter, Escherichia, Hafnia, Klebsiella, Salmonella, Serratia, Shigella.*

NEGATIVE IN: Groups of *Proteus, Providence.*

PLEURAL FLUID CULTURE

SYNONYM: Lung Fluid Culture, Paracentesis Thoracis Culture.

NURSES' RESPONSIBILITY:

It is the responsibility of the nurse to assist the physician in obtaining the pleural fluid and to transport the fluid to the laboratory *immediately* upon collection. The fluid must be placed in a sterile container and kept free from contamination at all times.

The fluid must be collected via sterile syringe with a large aspirating needle (16 gauge) under rigid aseptic conditions by thoracentesis (paracentesis thoracis). The patient should be instructed to sit upright, leaning forward with his arms raised and his hands on opposite shoulders. The skin must be cleansed and prepared as for any minor surgical procedure. The physician will select the area of greatest dullness and the puncture will be made. If the selected point is the sixth or seventh interspace, the puncture will be made at the midaxillary line; if it is the eighth interspace, the puncture will be made below the angle of the scapula.

Pleural fluid, when aspirated, is inoculated onto the various selective media in an attempt to isolate any organisms which may be the causative agents of the inflammation. The fluid may be centrifuged at a high speed for 20 to 30 minutes, the supernatant fluid poured off and discarded. The sediment is then used for the cultures and a Gram stain (see p. 59).

Among the more common selective media used for pleural fluid growth are blood agar, eosin methylene blue media, glucose agar slant, tryptose broth, and thioglycollate glucose broth. If a *Hemophilus* organism is suspected, a streak of *Staphylococcus aureus* organisms may be added to the blood agar plate to provide the necessary factor for Factor V growth. If tuberculosis is suspected, a stain is usually made by means of the Ziehl-Neelsen method (p. 7), and the material is cultured for *Mycobacterium tuberculosis* (p. 99). If a fungus growth is suspected, additional culture media and tests must be run (see *Fungus Culture,* p. 129).

The media which has been inoculated with the fluid is incubated at 37°C and observed for morphological and cultural characteristics at 24 and 48 hours.

78

SPECIMEN REQUIRED:

A few milliliters of sterile pleural fluid are needed.

PRESERVATIVE:

None is required. However, if the fluid is not cultured immediately, it must be refrigerated at 4 to 6°C until used.

LENGTH OF TIME REQUIRED TO PERFORM TEST:

A minimum of 24 to 48 hours should be allowed.

NORMAL VALUES: No pathogens isolated.

POSITIVE IN:

Infections caused by *Diplococcus pneumoniae, Hemophilus influenzae, Mycobacterium tuberculosis, Staphylococcus aureus, Streptococcus pyogenes,* others.

POTASSIUM CYANIDE TEST FOR BACTERIAL IDENTIFICATION

SYNONYM: KCN Test.

NURSES' RESPONSIBILITY:

No special preparation of the patient is needed.

PRINCIPLE OF THE TEST:

Certain organisms, such as those of groups *Aerobacter* and *Proteus,* possess the ability to grow in a potassium cyanide broth, while others do not possess this characteristic. The test is useful in differentiating organisms of the groups *Salmonella* and *Shigella* from the Enterobacteriaceae. The test is recorded as:

Growth in KCN Broth: Positive.

No Growth in KCN Broth: Negative.

SPECIMEN REQUIRED: A few colonies of the test organisms are needed.

PRESERVATIVE: None is permitted.

LENGTH OF TIME REQUIRED TO PERFORM TEST:

A minimum of eight to twelve hours following growth of the initial culture must be allowed.

POSITIVE IN:

Groups of *Aerobacter, Citrobacter, Hafnia, Klebsiella, Proteus, Providencia, Serratia.*

NEGATIVE IN:

Groups of *Arizona, Escherichia, Salmonella, Shigella.*

QUELLUNG REACTION

SYNONYMS: Neufeld's Test, Capsular Swelling Test for Pneumo-cocci.

NURSES' RESPONSIBILITY:

No special preparation of the patient is needed.

PRINCIPLE OF THE TEST:

When type-specific antibody previously obtained from rabbits is added to certain types of encapsulated pneumocci, the capsule enlarges or "swells" in a matter of a few minutes, indicating the serological type of pneumococcus.

Groups A through F pneumococci sera are each added to a few colonies of the test organism in saline and the reaction observed for swelling under the oil immersion objective of the microscope. If desired, the test may be performed directly on fresh sputum, spinal fluid, nasopharyngeal mucus or other materials.

The test may be performed with other encapsulated organisms, although the test is most frequently used for the pneumococcus.

This test is seldom used today, as treatment for pneumococcal infections is not dependent upon determination of the specific capsular type. However, since the test may be used for other organisms, it has been included in this book. The test is significant in that the pneumococcus or other organisms may be identified *directly* from test material in only a short time.

SPECIMEN REQUIRED:

A small aliquot of the test material (24-hour pneumococcal culture, sputum, spinal fluid, blood, nasopharyngeal mucus) is needed.

PRESERVATIVE: None is permitted.

LENGTH OF TIME REQUIRED TO PERFORM TEST:

A minimum of 15 minutes should be allowed.

NORMAL VALUES: There are no set normal values for this test.

POSITIVE IN:

Type-specific pneumococcal infections, few other organisms.

SENSITIVITY STUDIES (BACTERIAL)

SYNONYM: Antibiotic Susceptibility Test.

NURSES' RESPONSIBILITY:

The specimen must be brought to the laboratory immediately upon collection. If the test is not performed at once, the specimen *must* be refrigerated.

PRINCIPLE OF THE TEST:

The bacterial sensitivity test is used to determine the effectiveness of chemotherapy. It tells the physician whether a particular antibiotic will be of any value in the treatment of the current infection. Since it is highly important that the patient not be overloaded with antibiotics, it is necessary to determine the most important antibiotic for treatment. There are several widely used methods of sensitivity studies, including the *agar diffusion serial tube dilution method,* and the *agar dilution method.* The most frequently used is the agar diffusion method. This employs commercially prepared discs or strips impregnated with known amounts of chemotherapeutic substances. Either the isolated organism from a pure culture or a direct specimen is uniformly inoculated onto a blood agar plate or other medium of choice and the discs placed upon the surface of the agar culture medium. After 24 hours incubation at 37°C, the test is examined for zones of inhibition of growth around the discs, each of which contains a chemotherapeutic substance. The test is usually read as diameter in millimeters of the zones of growth inhibition. For example, a high degree of sensitivity may be indicated by a large zone of inhibition around the "low" concentration of the antibacterial substance, even though the zone of the "high" concentration is lesser in diameter. The test is, therefore, read as a function of the rate of diffusion of activity into the culture medium. A high and low concentration may be used, which are related to the blood level maintained by an average dosage of the drug.

In the Kirby-Bauer method of disc sensitivity testing, zone diameters are measured using the template or zone measuring chart. The plate containing the sensitivity discs is placed over the zone measuring chart, and the zone on the plate is compared to the zones on the tabs. The zone diameter is read after six to fourteen hours incubation.

There are several advantages to this method; it is (1) simple, (2) less expensive, (3) less time-consuming, and (4) reliable.

Generally speaking, the gram-positive bacteria are sensitive to penicillin and the gram-negative bacteria to streptomycin. However, exceptions occur and certain kinds of bacteria vary widely in their sensitivity to antibacterial chemotherapeutic agents. Therefore, sensitivity studies of isolates may be run routinely in some laboratories.

SPECIMEN REQUIRED:

Any specimen containing bacteria may be used for sensitivity studies. This includes specimens such as feces, urine, abscesses, wounds, and blood.

PRESERVATIVE: None is permitted.

LENGTH OF TIME REQUIRED TO PERFORM TEST:

A minimum of 24 hours should be allowed.

NORMAL VALUES:

Sensitive: Distinct zone of inhibition around disc(s) of one or more antibiotics.

SIGNIFICANCE OF FINDINGS: Refer to *Principle of the Test.*

SINUS CULTURE

The patient should be made comfortable while the rhinologist obtains the material from the sinuses. A good source of illumination is necessary during the entire examination.

The material is obtained by means of a sterile swab, and is returned to the sterile tube (containing a transport medium) from which it was originally taken. Failure to transport the specimen to the laboratory for culture immediately after the collection may result in an unsatisfactory bacteriological examination, since certain pathogens are very fragile and tend to die under adverse conditions.

Principle of the Test:

Material from the sinuses is cultured in an attempt to isolate any pathogenic organisms which may be present.

The swab containing the material is used to inoculate the differential plate media and the clock-streak method of isolation used.

Cultures are made both aerobically and anaerobically, or in a 10% carbon dioxide atmosphere. The differential media most frequently used in the isolation of pathogens from a sinus culture include blood agar, eosin methylene blue (EMB), chocolate agar, MacConkey agar, Salmonella-Shigella agar (SS), thioglycollate broth, and brain-heart infusion broth. Cultures may also be made for fungal growth and viral growth if the physician deems it necessary.

Specimen Required:

One or two swabs containing the material obtained from the sinus.

Preservative: None is permitted.

Length of Time Required to Perform Test:

A minimum of 24 to 48 hours should be allowed.

Normal Values: No pathogens isolated.

ABNORMAL FINDINGS:

Pathogens that may be isolated from sinus cultures include *Aspergillus* sp., *Bacillus subtilis, Corynebacterium diptheriae, Diplococcus pneumoniae, Hemophilus influenzae, Klebsiella pneumoniae, Neisseria meningitidis, Proteus* spp. *Pseudomonas aeruginosa, Staphylococcus* spp., *Streptococcus* spp.

SPUTUM (ROUTINE)

The patient should be instructed to rinse his mouth thoroughly before the collection in order to avoid contamination from food particles and other normal mouth inhabitants.

The morning sputum or a 24-hour collection is best for a routine examination. The patient must be instructed to cough deeply from the lungs rather than a shallow cough which may result in mere saliva. In cases of tuberculosis, there may be times when there is little or no sputum. In such cases, aspiration of the stomach may be essential to obtain material that has been swallowed. Since infants and very young children have a tendency to swallow the sputum, an examination of the feces may be of some value. The patient must be instructed to avoid smearing the sputum; all precautions should be taken not to infect personnel.

The container most suitable for such a collection is a sterile, wide-mouthed bottle with a screw cap. sufficient to hold the entire amount. Paper containers should not be used at any time. The container must be kept covered at all times to avoid contamination. If contamination with sputum occurs, the patient's bedstand and other room furnishings must be cleansed immediately with disinfectant.

PRINCIPLE OF THE TEST:

The routine examination of sputum should include the following:

1. *Volume:* A general idea as to the volume expectorated in a certain length of time (i.e. 24 hours) is essential since in some diseases, such as incipient tuberculosis or pulmonary edema, the quantity is very minute, while in diseases such as empyema or lung abscess it may be excessively large. It is not necessary to measure the sputum accurately but rather to obtain a general idea of the volume. The volume of the sputum expectorated tends to serve as an index of the prognosis.

2. *Color:* The color of the sputum is a necessary part of the routine examination. It tells the physician a great deal concerning the composition of the specimen. For example, if the sputum

contains *red streaks,* it most likely contains blood which strongly suggests tuberculosis. An *orange to rusty* colored sputum may indicate lobar pneumonia or decomposed hemoglobin. A *yellowish-green* sputum is strongly suggestive of chronic bronchitis or advanced tuberculosis, while a *bright green* sputum is found in jaundice and lobar pneumonia. A *brown* color suggests hematin, while a *reddish tint* may indicate the color of iron oxide. A *grayish to black* color may be caused by hematemesis, coal dust, or carbon.

3. *Consistency and Appearance:* The sputum is usually classified according to the consistency (tenacity) of the specimen, which may be recorded as mucopurulent, seropurulent, purulent, bloody, mucoid, or serous. The report concerning the consistency and appearance should accompany the color description. For example, the sputum would be described as "colorless and serous."

4. *Odor:* Normally, fresh and undecomposed sputum will have no odor. Varying kinds of odors may occur, such as sour, putrid, sweet, or cheese-like which may be found in conditions such as lung abscesses, gangrene and tuberculosis, and bronchiectasis.

5. *Reaction:* Fresh sputum is normally alkaline. However, in certain conditions in which the sputum has been in the lung for a long period of time, the reaction may be acid.

6. *Layer Formation (Stratification):* In certain diseases, such as bronchiectasis, gangrene, and lung abscess, the sputum separates into *three* distinct layers upon allowing it to stand in a large cylinder. The three layers are a frothy layer on top, a clear middle layer, and a bottom layer containing cellular elements and the dense mucus.

7. *Microscopic Examination:* This should include the following:

Unstained Smear: A carefully selected drop of sputum should be transferred to a clean slide and coverslipped. The slide is then examined under the low-and high-power objectives of the microscope for the following structures:

Crystals, such as Charcot-Leyden, cholesterol,
  leucine, tyrosine, inorganic salts, fatty
  acids.
Pus cells (white blood cells).
Erythrocytes (red blood cells).
Elastic fibers.
Curschmann's spirals.
Myelin globules.
Pigmented cells, such as "heart/failure" or
  dust cells.
Bronchial casts.
Molds, fungi, and yeast.
Mucus.
Animal parasites.

Stained Smear: A carefully selected drop of sputum is spread on a clean glass slide and smeared such as a drop of blood for the differential. A Wright's stain is used to stain the slide after the sputum has been allowed to dry and the slide flamed.

Six kinds of leukocytes may be found and are recorded in percentages. The slide is examined for the following:

Polymorphonuclear leukocytes.
Lymphocytes.
Eosinophils.
Monocytes.
Basophils.
Band cells.
Erythrocytes.
Epithelial cells.

A Gram stain (see p. 59) is employed for the study of bacteria.
The sputum may also be carefully examined for any other structures which might be present, either by macroscopic or microscopic examination.

SPECIMEN REQUIRED:

A small quantity (1.0 to 2.0 ml) of freshly expectorated sputum is needed, or a 24-hour specimen if the total output is to be measured.

PRESERVATIVE:

No preservative should be added, since it would tend to distort or destroy certain structures. The sputum should be refrigerated until the tests can be performed.

LENGTH OF TIME REQUIRED TO PERFORM TEST:

A minimum of two hours should be allowed for this testing—with the exception of cultures, whch required 24 hours to eight weeks for completion.

NORMAL FINDINGS:

A few pus cells, erythrocytes, bacteria, and mucus threads, as well as a few squamous epithelial cells, are considered normal constituents of sputum. Nonpathogenic yeasts, molds, and diphtheroids may be present as contaminants. Myelin globules are insignificant.

ABNORMAL FINDINGS:

Pathological findings not discussed previously in this section include the causative organisms found in the sputum and their respective diseases.

1. *Animal Parasites:* Ascaridiasis *(Ascaris lumbricoides)*, hookworm disease *(Ancylostoma duodenale* or *Necator americanus)*, lung fluke infestation *(Paragonimus westermani)*, strongyloidiasis *(Strongyloides stercoralis)*.

2. *Bacteria:* Bubonic plague *(Pasteurella pestis)*, influenza *(Hemophilus influenzae)*, pneumonia *(Klebsiella pneumoniae, Diplococcus pneumoniae, Staphylococcus aureus,* or *Streptococcus pyogenes)*, tuberculosis *(Mycobacterium tuberculosis)*.

3. *Bronchial casts:* Diphtheria, lobar pneumonia, chronic plastic bronchitis.

4. *Charcot-Leyden crystals:* Bronchial asthma.

5. *Curshmann's spirals:* Bronchial asthma.

6. *Dittrich's plugs:* Bronchiectasis.

7. *Eosinophils:* Bronchial asthma.

8. *Elastic fibers:* Abscess of the lung, gangrene of the lung, tuberculosis.

9. *Fungi:* Candidiasis *(Candida albicans)* cryptococcus *(Cryptococcus neoformans)*, histoplasmosis *(Histoplasma capsulatum)*, sporotrichosis *(Sporotrichum schenckii)*, others.

10. *Heart failure cells:* Long-standing pulmonary congestion due to heart failure.

11. *Lung stones:* Chronic tuberculosis.

12. *Molds* and *yeasts:* Coccidioides granuloma *(Coccidioidal immitis)*, pulmonary blastomycosis *(Blastomyces dermatitidis)*.

13. *Pigmented cells:* Pulmonary infarction, pulmonary hemorrhage.

14. *Red Blood Cells:* Bronchiectasis, tuberculosis.

SPUTUM (ROUTINE CULTURE)

NURSES' RESPONSIBILITY:
The instructions for the collection of the specimen are discussed under *Sputum (Routine)*, page 86.

PRINCIPLE OF THE TEST:
The culture is used to isolate any bacteria which may be present in the specimen. A sputum culture is frequently treated as a lung culture.

The suspected disease process and, consequently, the organism play an important role in the selection of the media onto which the sputum is inoculated. Generally, the media of choice in sputum cultures include blood agar, eosin methylene blue (EMB), tellurite, Staph 110, phenol alcohol (PA), thioglycollate, and tryptose broth. Various other media are frequently used.

A small loopful of the specimen is inoculated onto the petri dish and streaked in a clocklike thinning motion. Broth and thioglycollate are also inoculated by means of a platinum wire. The media are incubated for 24 to 48 hours at 37°C and examined for the growth. Identification of the organisms is made by employing Gram, methylene blue, and Giemsa stains.

SPECIMEN REQUIRED:
One or two milliliters of a freshly expectorated sputum are needed.

PRESERVATIVE: None is permitted.

LENGTH OF TIME REQUIRED TO PERFORM TEST:
A minimum of 24 to 48 hours should be allowed. Cultures of sputum for *Mycobacterium tuberculosis* take considerably longer.

NORMAL VALUES: No pathogenic organisms isolated.

ABNORMAL FINDINGS:
Pathogens that may be isolated from a sputum culture include *Actinobacillus mallei, Aspergillus fumigatus, Bacillus anthracis, Bordetella pertussis, Borrelia vincentii, Brucella melitensis, Candida albicans, Coccidiodes immitis, Corynebacterium diphtheriae, Diplococcus pneumoniae, Eberthella typhosa, Escherichia coli,*

Gaffkya tetragena, Geotrichum candidum, Hemophilus influenzae, Histoplasma capsulatum, Klebsiella pneumoniae, Neisseria catarrhalis, N. intracellularis, Nocardia asteroides, Pasteurella pestis, Proteus vulgaris, Pseudomonas aeruginosa, Shigella dysenteriae, Staphylococcus aureus (coagulase positive), *Streptococcus pyogenes.*

SYNOVIAL FLUID COLLECTION

Synonym: Joint Fluid Collection.

Nurses' Responsibility:

The puncture may be performed in an operating room, but is usually done in the patient's room. *It is essential* that all materials necessary for the puncture be kept sterile. A table should be covered with sterile towels. Materials needed for the puncture vary, depending upon the person performing the procedure. A typical sterile collection tray should be set up and contain the following items:

1 (ea.) 2 ml syringe.
1 (ea.) 10 ml syringe.
1 (ea.) 20 ml syringe.
1 (ea.) 50 ml syringe.
2 (ea.) 25 g x $\frac{5}{8}$ inch needles.
2 (ea.) 20 g x $1\frac{1}{2}$ inch needles.
2 (ea.) 18 g x $1\frac{1}{2}$ inch needles.
2 medicine glasses.
Sterile test tubes, complete with tight fitting caps (one containing an anticoagulant).
Cotton balls.
Forceps.
4 prep sponges.
3 towels.
Drape with $2\frac{1}{2}$ inch hole.
Gloves, sizes 8 and 9.
Ethyl chloride in a pressurized can, or 2% procaine hydrochloride.

The procedure should be explained to the patient prior to beginning in order to alleviate apprehension. Sterile technique must be employed since this is a surgical technique. The skin is cleansed thoroughly with soap and water and then with iodine and alcohol. The towels are draped to keep the area sterile, and the drape placed over the area.

The proposed site of puncture is anesthetized with either procaine hydrochloride or ethyl chloride. Although the knee is the most frequent source of fluid, it may also be obtained from other joints such as swollen shoulders, ankles, or hips. In obtaining fluid from the knee, it may be aspirated from the suprapatellar bursa —entering about two inches above the patella—or it may be obtained from the cavity.

As soon as the anesthesia is effective, the needle is inserted and as much fluid as possible aspirated. The fluid is placed in tubes suitable for the needs of the various tests. Refer to the specific tests for instructions concerning handling of the specimens.

The patient should have a bandage placed over the site of the puncture as soon as the needle is removed. It usually is not necessary for him to remain in a resting state following the aspiration.

SYNOVIAL FLUID CULTURE

Synonym: Joint Fluid Culture.

Nurses' Responsibility:

It is the responsibility of the nurse to assist the physician in the aspiration of the synovial fluid (refer to *Synovial Fluid Collection,* p. 93)

Principle of the Test:

Isolation of any pathogenic organism which may be present is demonstrated by inoculating a loopful of synovial fluid onto the media of choice for the suspected organisms; the clock-streak method of isolation is used.

The media of choice for isolation of organisms in synovial fluid includes thioglycollate glucose broth, blood agar (aerobic and anaerobic), and chocolate agar. Cultures are incubated in an atmosphere of 10% carbon dioxide for best results.

Specimen Required: A few drops of synovial fluid are needed.

Preservative: None is permitted.

Length of Time Required to Perform Test:

A minimum of 24 to 48 hours should be allowed.

Normal Values: No organisms isolated.

Significance of Findings:

The organisms may be either blood-born or spread from soft tissue or bone lesions. Pathogenic bacteria most often isolated from synovial fluid include *Diplococcus pneumoniae, Neisseria gonorrhoeae, N. meningitidis, Mycobacterium tuberculosis,* PPLO (pleuropneumonia-like organisms), *Staphylococcus aureus, Streptococcus pyogenes.*

THROAT AND NASOPHARYNGEAL CULTURE

NURSES' RESPONSIBILITY:

The throat and nasopharyngeal specimens are obtained by means of either a cotton-tipped swab or an alginate swab.

The *throat culture* is made by "swabbing" material from the inflamed area. The tongue is depressed by means of a wooden tongue depressor, while the swab is carefully inserted into the mouth. Extreme care must be taken to avoid touching the oral surface, tongue, or the cheek. The swab is vigorously rubbed over the inflamed area in obtaining the material.

The *nasopharyngeal culture* is obtained by means of a special nasopharyngeal swab of light aluminum or copper wire. This culture is much preferred over the throat and nose culture since less contaminants are encountered. The swab is inserted through the nasal passage, rotating as it is inserted. The swab is placed in a sterile container, containing Stuart's transport medium or other similar medium, and taken to the laboratory *immediately,* since certain pathogens, such as *Neisseria meningitidis,* tend to die under adverse conditions.

In certain cases, two or three swabs may be needed—one for the culture and two for the smears. If in doubt, the laboratory or attending physician should be consulted.

PRINCIPLE OF THE TEST:

Inflammatory tissue is cultured in an attempt to isolate any pathogenic organisms of the mouth and nose (nasopharynx) which may be present.

The swab containing the material is rubbed onto the differential plate media. The selective media most frequently used in the isolation of pathogens from the throat and nose are blood agar, eosin methylene blue (EMB), MacConkey agar, thioglycollate, and tryptose broth. In suspected cases of diphtheria, additional media may be inoculated. This often includes a cystine blood tellurite agar plate, Tinsdale medium, Loeffler's serum slant, and other similar media. All throat and nasopharyngeal cultures are incubated at 37°C anaerobically in 10% carbon dioxide atmosphere for 18 to 24 hours, as well as aerobically, and observed for morphological and cultural characteristics at 18, 24, and 48 hours. The growth on tellurite appears as typically smooth, grayish-black convex colonies.

In possible cases of Vincent's angina, the swab is rolled across a glass slide, stained with methylene blue, and examined for the characteristic organisms.

Some microbiologists prefer to use the "pour plate" method for isolating organisms of the nasopharynx. The organisms are allowed to grow in a broth culture for four to six hours. One loopful of the culture is inoculated into a melted blood agar-sterile citrate blood mixture. This mixture is poured into a sterile petri dish and observed for characteristic growth.

SPECIMEN REQUIRED: Refer to *Nurses' Responsibility* for collection.

PRESERVATIVE: None is permitted.

LENGTH OF TIME REQUIRED TO PERFORM TEST:
A minimum of 24 to 48 hours should be allowed.

NORMAL VALUES:
No pathogens isolated. Normal flora may be present in the mouth and are of no significance unless found in excessive numbers. Among the organisms found in a normal throat are *Aerobacter aerogenes, Escherichia coli, Hemophilus hemolyticus, Proteus* spp., *Neisseria catarrhalis, Staphylococcus epidermis, Streptococcus viridans.*

PATHOLOGICAL FINDINGS:
Bordetella pertussis, Borrelia vincentii, B. bussalis, Candida albicans (predominance), *Corynebacterium diphtheriae, Diplococcus pneumoniae, Hemophilus influenzae, Neisseria meningitidis, Staphylococcus aureus* (coagulase positive), *Streptococcus pyogenes* (group A, occasionally groups B, C, and G), *Treponema microdentium,* others.

TRIPHENYL TETRAZOLIUM CHLORIDE TEST

SYNONYM: T.T.C. Test.

NURSES' RESPONSIBILITY:

In certain cases, the physician may wish the urine specimen to be sterile and request a catheterized specimen for the test. A physician's order for this procedure is essential. Since there is a great chance of accidental infection of the patient's bladder during catheterization, the utmost care in aseptic technique must be taken. In the cases of infants and younger children, small plastic containers may be fastened with adhesive tape over the penis of males, and the urethral meatus of females.

PRINCIPLE OF THE TEST:

This is a screening test for *significant* bacteriuria. An aliquot of the patient's urine is added to a small quantity of a working solution consisting of triphenyl tetrazolium chloride and saturated monobasic sodium phosphate. The mixture is incubated for six hours and is then examined for a macroscopic pink-red precipitate which indicates a *positive* reaction. A pink supernatant with no precipitate indicates a negative reaction. The test is most often positive in bacterial colony counts of more than 100,000 colonies per milliliter of urine.

SPECIMEN REQUIRED:

A few cubic centimeters of a random urine specimen or a catheterized urine specimen are needed.

PRESERVATIVE: None is permitted.

LENGTH OF TIME REQUIRED TO PERFORM TEST:

A minimum of six to eight hours should be allowed.

NORMAL VALUES: Negative.

POSITIVE IN:

Bacterial infections in which the colony count exceeds 100,000 /ml urine.

TUBERCULOSIS STUDY (SPUTUM)

SYNONYMS:

T.B. Study (Sputum), Acid-Fast Bacillus Study (Sputum), A.F.B. (Sputum), *Mycobacterium tuberculosis* Study (Sputum).

NURSES' RESPONSIBILITY:

The directions for the collection of the specimen are discussed under *Sputum (Routine),* page 86

PRINCIPLE OF THE TEST:

Several studies are of value in the examination of sputum for tuberculosis. Among these are the direct smear, culture, animal inoculation, and fluorescent antibody.

1. *Direct Smear:* A preparation of the sputum is made by smearing the specimen between two glass slides and fixing with a Bunsen burner by flaming the slide. The slides are stained by means of an acid-fast staining technique. Among the more popular at the present time are the *Ziehl-Neelsen method* and the *Gross "cold" method,* the latter requiring no heating. Acid-fast organisms stain red, while other organisms stain blue. The finding of acid-fast organisms does not, however, verify tuberculosis as the disease, since some nonpathogenic acid-fast organisms may also be present in the sputum. Therefore, further verification must be made by culture, animal inoculation, or fluorescent antibody.

2. *Tuberculosis Culture:* The sputum must be liquified since a liquid state often reveals the tuberculosis organisms, whereas a direct smear may not. Sodium hydroxide is the most common liquifying reagent, although sodium hypochlorite and trisodium phosphate may also be used. The liquefaction process also destroys bacteria other than acid-fast organisms, preventing overgrowth or toxic effects to the experimental animal. *Lowenstein-Jensen, Petragnani* Middlebrook 7H10, or some other media similar to these is recommended for this type of culture.

A sterile swab is used to spread the sputum over the slant of the media. The slanted tubes are incubated at 37°C for 24 hours and examined.

If negative, they are reincubated for three to eight weeks, with periodic examination for the acid-fast organisms.

3. *Animal Inoculation.* The sputum should be liquified as described under tuberculosis culture. Two guinea pigs are most often used since one may die due to toxic effects before the test is completed. A quantity of 0.1 to 0.5 ml of the liquified sputum is injected subcutaneously into the groin of the guinea pigs. It may also be injected intramuscularly or intraperitoneally, since there appears to be no difference in the number of positive cases with any of these three routes of injection. A suspension of the growth obtained by culture may be injected for conclusive diagnosis.

At the end of six weeks, an autopsy is performed on the animals and examination is made for the tubercular lesions. Slides for the tuberculosis organism are made from the various infected organs.

4. *Fluorescent Antibody:* A small quantity of either the freshly expectorated sputum or a culture is placed in the well of a slide designed for fluorescent antibody work. The slide is immersed in a Coplin jar containing acetone or some other fixing agent and is allowed to "fix" at −20°C for four hours. The slide is then stained by one of four methods: direct, inhibition, indirect, or complement staining. Refer to *Fluorescent Antibody Test,* page 52 for further descriptions of these staining techniques.

SPECIMEN REQUIRED:

A small quantity of freshly expectorated sputum in a sterile container is needed.

PRESERVATIVE: None is permitted.

LENGTH OF TIME REQUIRED TO PERFORM TEST:

A minimum of one hour should be allowed for the direct smear, four to eight weeks for the culture, six to eight weeks for the animal inoculation, and five to six hours for the fluorescent antibody.

NORMAL VALUES:

No acid-fast bacilli characteristic of *Mycobacterium tuberculosis* seen or isolated.

PATHOLOGICAL FINDINGS:

The above tests are found in infections caused by *Mycobacterium tuberculosis.*

TYN TEST

SYNONYM: Trichomonas, Yeast *(Candida albicans),* and *Neisseria* Test.

These individual tests are used in the diagnosis of vaginal infections. The three essential and separate tests include *T. vaginalis* (a one-cell parasite), yeast *(C. albicans),* and *N. gonorrhoeae* (a bacterium causing gonorrhea in man).

These three tests are described individually in this book, and the reader may find them listed as follows:

Candida Identification, page 122.

Neisseria Gonorrhoeae Tests, page 67.

Trichomonas Vaginalis Test, page 226.

UREA TEST

SYNONYM: Christiansen's Urea Test.

NURSES' RESPONSIBILITY:

No special preparation of the patient is needed.

PRINCIPLE OF THE TEST:

Certain bacteria, such as *Proteus* species, hydrolyze urea rapidly, releasing ammonia, which in turn imparts a red color to the test medium.

A few colonies of the test organism are inoculated into urea medium, incubated at 37°C, and the color reaction observed at two, four, and twenty-four hours. The test is read as follows:

Pink-red: Positive.

No Color Change: Negative.

The test is often employed in differentiating *Proteus* from *Salmonella* and *Shigella* species.

SPECIMEN REQUIRED: A few colonies of the test organism are needed.

PRESERVATIVE: None is permitted.

LENGTH OF TIME REQUIRED TO PERFORM TEST:

A minimum of two to twenty-four hours following growth of the organism should be allowed.

NORMAL VALUES: There are no set normal values for this test.

POSITIVE IN:

Aerobacter spp., *Klebsiella* spp., *Pasteurella* spp., *Proteus* spp., *Serratia* spp., few others.

NEGATIVE IN: *Salmonella* spp., *Shigella* spp., others.

URINE CULTURE (QUALITATIVE)

SYNONYMS: Ua Culture, Ur Culture.

NURSES' RESPONSIBILITY:

It is imperative that urine for bacteriological examination be free of contamination. Since there is a great chance of accidental infection of the patient's bladder during catheterization, the utmost care in aseptic technique must be taken. In many cases, a "clean voided" urine may be used for the culture.

In the cases of infants and younger children, small plastic containers may be fastened with adhesive tape over the penis of males, and the urethral meatus of females.

In suspected cases of diseases such as tuberculosis of the kidney, special methods and times of collection may be required. The laboratory will be able to furnish the necessary details for these tests.

In all cases, the urine must be transported to the laboratory immediately following the collection. If immediate culture of the urine is not possible, the specimen must be kept at refrigerator temperature of 4° to 6°C until cultured within 24 hours.

PRINCIPLE OF THE TEST:

The urine is cultured in an attempt to isolate any pathogenic organisms which may be present. A small amount of the uncentrifuged urine is inoculated onto differential media, such as blood agar and eosin methylene blue agar (EMB).

The differential media most often used in the isolation of pathogens from a urine culture are blood agar, EMB, trypticase soy broth, and thioglycollate broth. Cultures may also be made for fungal growth (see *Fungus Culture,* p. 129) and viral growth (see *Virus Culture,* p. 182) if the physician deems it necessary.

The plates are incubated aerobically and in a 10% carbon dioxide atmosphere at 37°C and are examined at 24 and 48 hours for cultural and morphological characteristics.

SPECIMEN REQUIRED:

Refer to *Nurses' Responsibility* for specimens and collections.

PRESERVATIVE:

None is permitted. If it is impossible to immediately culture the urine, it must be refrigerated.

LENGTH OF TIME REQUIRED TO PERFORM TEST:

A period of 24 to 48 hours should be allowed.

NORMAL VALUES: No pathogens isolated.

ABNORMAL FINDINGS:

Pathogens that may be isolated from a urine culture include *Alcaligenes fecalis, Diplococcus pneumoniae, Escherichia coli, Neisseria gonorrhoeae, Proteus* spp., *Pseudomonas aeruginosa, Salmonella* spp., *Shigella* spp., *Staphylococcus aureus* (coagulase positive) , *Streptococcus* spp.

URINE CULTURE (QUANTITATIVE)

SYNONYM: Colony Count (Urine)

NURSES' RESPONSIBILITY: Refer to *Urine Culture (Qualitative)*, page 103.

PRINCIPLE OF THE TEST:

The urine is cultured, using a standard inoculating loop (4 mm and delivering 0.01 ml), in an attempt to enumerate the number of bacterial colonies present in the sample. Different dilutions of the urine are used in deep-pour cultures to facilitate quantitation.

The number of colonies counted on the bacteriological media plate is multiplied by the factor 100 to determine the number of organisms present. Normally, there are less than 10,000 colonies per milliliter of urine. However in bacterial infections of the urinary tract, the count may rise to 100,000/ml urine. In these cases, various dilutions of the urine in sterile saline are made. The dilutions are usually 1:1,000 and 1:100,000. The number of colonies are counted by means of a colony counter or some other suitable means of colony counting.

SPECIMEN REQUIRED:

A few drops of a sterile urine specimen. Refer to *Nurses' Responsibility, Urine Culture (Qualitative)*, page 103.

PRESERVATIVE:

None is permitted. If immediate culture of the urine is not possible, the specimen must be kept at refrigerated temperature of 4° to 6°C until cultured within 24 hours.

LENGTH OF TIME REQUIRED TO PERFORM TEST:

Results are usually attained within 24 hours; however, it may take as long as 48 hours.

NORMAL VALUES: Less than 100 colonies per milliliter urine.

INCREASED IN:

Colony counts may be increased in bacterial infections caused by such pathogens as *Alcaligenes fecalis, Diplococcus pneumoniae,*

Escherichia coli, Neisseria gonorrhoeae, Proteus spp., *Pseudomonas aeruginosa, Salmonella* spp., *Shigella* spp., *Streptococcus* spp., others.

VOGES - PROSKAUER TEST

SYNONYM: Acetoin Color Test.

NURSES' RESPONSIBILITY:

No special preparation of the patient is needed.

PRINCIPLE OF THE TEST:

Upon the addition of an alkali such as potassium hydroxide, acetylmethylcarbinol is oxidized to diacetyl by the action of various bacteria that have been previously cultured in a buffered peptone dextrose broth for 24 to 48 hours. The reagent is added to the culture, and the tube is incubated at both 37°C and room temperature, each for four hours, with occasional mixing. The formed diacetyl combines with the guanidine radical of creatine to form a pink dye compound.

This qualitative test is employed most often in the differentiation of *Escherichia coli* and *Aerobacter cloacae*. The test is reported as follows:

Pink Color: V-P positive.

Colorless: V-P negative.

SPECIMEN REQUIRED: A few colonies of the test organism are needed.

PRESERVATIVE: None is permitted.

NORMAL VALUES: There are no set normal values for this test.

LENGTH OF TIME REQUIRED TO PERFORM TEST:

Approximately 24 to 48 hours from the beginning of the test culture are needed.

POSITIVE IN:

Aerobacter cloacae, Klebsiella pneumoniae, Proteus spp. (some), few others.

NEGATIVE IN:

Escherichia coli, E. freundii, Providence spp., *Salmonella* spp., *Shigella* spp., others.

WOUND CULTURE

Nurses' Responsibility:

The surface area surrounding the wound must be cleansed with an antiseptic solution, such as alcohol or iodine. The material is obtained by gently touching the clean inner tissue of the wound with a sterile swab. The swab is returned to the original sterile tube from which it was taken, and transported to the laboratory without delay. Failure to transport the specimen immediately upon collection may result in an unsatisfactory bacteriological examination.

Principle of the Test:

Material from a wound is cultured in an attempt to isolate any pathogenic organisms which may be present. The swab containing the material is rubbed onto the differential plate. Cultures must be made both aerobically and anaerobically. For anaerobiosis, the cultures are most often incubated in "an atmosphere" jar such as the Brewer jar, whereby the oxygen is depleted by means of electrically heated, platinized asbestos. A simpler and much safer method of anaerobic culturing is use of the Gaspak jar. In this method, an anaerobic atmosphere is created when hydrogen is produced by the Gaspak envelope reacting with oxygen in the presence of the catalyst.

The selective media most often used in the isolation of pathogens from a wound are blood agar, eosin methylene blue (EMB), MacConkey agar, Salmonella-Shigella (SS), thioglycollate broth, and brain-heart infusion broth. Cultures may also be made for fungal growth (see *Fungus Culture,* p. 129) and viral growth (see *Virus Culture,* p. 182) if the physician deems it necessary.

Specimen Required: Refer to *Nurses' Responsibility.*

Preservative: None is permitted.

Length of Time Required to Perform Test:

A minimum of 24 to 48 hours should be allowed.

Normal Values: No pathogens isolated.

Abnormal Findings:

Pathogens which may be isolated from wound cultures include

Clostridium perfringens, C. tetani, Corynebacterium diphtheriae, Neisseria meningitidis, Staphylococcus aureus (coagulase positive), viruses such as those causing smallpox and herpes, others.

REFERENCES

Anderson, W.A.D.: *Pathology*, 5th ed. St. Louis, C.V. Mosby, 1966.

Baker, Francis Joseph, Silverton, R.E., and Luckcock, E.D.: *Introduction to Medical Laboratory Technology*, 4th ed. London, Butterworth's, 1966.

Bailey, W., and Scott, Elvyn G.: *Diagnostic Bacteriology*, 2nd ed. St. Louis, C.V. Mosby, 1966.

Bailey, W., and Scott, Elvyn G.: *Diagnostic Bacteriology*. St. Louis, C.V. Mosby, 1962.

Beaver, William C.: *General Biology; The Science of Biology*. St. Louis, C.V. Mosby, 1962.

Bisset, K.A.: *The Cytology and Life-History of Bacteria*, 3rd ed. Edinburgh and London, E. and E. Livingstone, 1970.

Blair, J.E., and Carr, M.: The bacteriophage typing of staphylococci. *J Infect Dis, 93:*1, 1953.

Boyd, William: *An Introduction to the Study of Medicine*, 5th ed. Philadelphia, Lea and Febiger, 1962.

Breed, Robert S., Murray, E.G.D., and Smith, Nathan R.: *Bergey's Manual of Determinative Bacteriology*, 7th ed. Baltimore, Williams and Wilkins, 1957.

Burdon, Kenneth L.: *Textbook of Microbiology*. New York, Macmillan, 1958.

Burrows, William: *Textbook of Microbiology*, 18th ed. Philadelphia and London, W.B. Saunders, 1963.

Cairns, J., Stent, G.S., and Watson, J.D.: *Phage and Origin of Molecular Biology*. New York, Cold Spring Harbor Laboratory of Quantitative Biology, 1966.

Chapman, J.: Human mycobacteriosis, *Med Sci 9:*555, 1961.

Coffee, J.M.: *Diagnostic Procedures and Reagents*, 3rd ed. Public Health Assoc., 1950.

Conn, H.J.: *Biological Stains*. Baltimore, Williams and Wilkins, 1961.

Conner, V., and Mallery, O.T., Jr.: Blood cultures. A clinical laboratory study of the methods. *Am J Clin Pathol, 21:*785, 1951.

Cooper, G.M., and Walter, A.W.: Application of the Neufeld reaction to the identification of types of pneumococci. *Am J Public Health, 25:*4, 1935.

Cummings, M.M.: The tubercle bacillus. Diagnostic procedures and reagents, 3rd ed. New York, Am. Public Health Assoc., 1950.

Damm, Henry C.: *Practical Manual for Clinical Laboratory Procedures*. Cleveland, Chemical Rubber Co., 1966.

Damm, Henry C.: *Handbook of Clinical Laboratory Data*. Cleveland, Chemical Rubber Co., 1965.

Davidsohn, Israel, and Wells, Benjamin B.: *Clinical Diagnosis by Laboratory Methods.* Philadelphia, W.B. Saunders, 1962.

Decancq, H. George, Jr., and Lee, Fred A.: *Mycoplasma pneumoniae. JAMA,* 1965.

Dienes, L.: Isolation of pleuropneumonia-like organisms from pathological specimens with the aid of penicillin. *Proc Soc Exp Biol Med, 64:*165, 1947.

Dowling, H.F.: *The Acute Bacterial Diseases, Their Diagnosis and Treatment.* Philadelphia, W.B. Saunders, 1948.

Dubos, Réne J.: *Bacterial and Mycotic Infections of Man,* 3rd ed. Philadelphia, J.B. Lippincott, 1958.

Edwards, P.R., and Ewing, W.H.: *Identification of Enterobacteriaceae.* Minneapolis, Burgess Publishing, 1955.

Eliot, C.P.: The Vi agglutination test as an aid in the detection of typhoid carriers. *Am J Hygiene, 31:*8, 1940.

Evans, Alice C.: Chronic brucellosis — the unreliability of diagnostic tests. *J Am Med Women's Assoc, 16:*942, 1961.

Fisk, R.T.: Studies on staphylococci. *J Infect Dis, 71:*153, 1942.

Francis, E., and Evans, A.C.: Agglutination, cross agglutination, and agglutinin adsorption in tularemia. *Public Health Rep, 41:*1273, 1926.

Frankel, Samm, Reitman, Stanley, and Sonnenwirth, Alex C.: *Gradwohl's Clinical Laboratory Methods and Diagnosis.* St. Louis, C.V. Mosby, 1963, Vol. I.

Frobisher, M., Jr.: *Fundamentals of Microbiology.* Philadelphia, W.B. Saunders, 1962.

Gibbs, B.M., and Skinner, F.A.: *Identification Methods for Microbiologists.* London, Academic Press, 1966.

Gillies, R.R., and Dodds, T.C.: *Bacteriology Illustrated.* Baltimore, Williams and Wilkins, 1968.

Grove, Donald C., and Randall, William A.: *Assay Methods of Antibiotics — A Laboratory Manual.* New York, Medical Encyclopedia, 1955.

Gruver, R.H., and Fries, E.D.: A study of diagnostic errors. *Ann Intern Med, 47:*108, 1957.

Harrison, T.R., Adams, Raymond D., Bennett, Ivan L., Resnik, W.H., Thorn, George W., and Wintrobe, M.M.: *Principles of Internal Medicine,* 5th ed. New York, McGraw-Hill, 1966.

Hull, T.G.: *Diseases Transmitted from Animals to Man.* Springfield, Thomas, 1954.

Jacobs, Morris B., Gerstein, Maurice J., and Walter, William G.: *Dictionary of Microbiology.* Princeton, Van Nostrand, 1957.

Jackson, G.G., Dowling, H.F., and Lepper, M.H.: Bacteriophage typing of staphylococci. II. Epidemiologic studies among patients, household contacts, and hospital personnel. *J Lab Clin Med, 44:*29, 1954.

Jordan, Edwin O., and Burrows, William: *Textbook of Bacteriology,* 13th ed. Philadelphia and London, W.B. Saunders, 1941.

Kass, E.H.: Bacteriuria and the diagnosis of infections of the urinary tract. *Arch Intern Med, 100:*709, 1957.

Kaufman, F.: *The Diagnosis of Salmonella Types.* Springfield, Thomas, 1950.

Kaufman, F.: *The Differentiation of Escherichia and Klebsiella Types.* Springfield, Thomas, 1951.

Kenny, George E., and Grayton, J. Thomas: Eaton pleuropneumonia-like organisms *(Mycoplasma pneumoniae)* complement-fixing antigen. *J Immunol, 95:*1, 1965.

Kerr, K.M., Mascoli, C.C., Alson, N.O., and Campbell, A.: Rapid and specific agglutination of Eaton Agent *(Mycoplasma pneumoniae). Am Soc Microbiol,* 1964.

Kimler, Alexander: *Manual of Clinical Bacteriology.* Philadelphia, J.B. Lippincott, 1961.

Kolmer, John A., Spaulding, Earle H., and Robinson, Howard W.: *Approved Laboratory Technic.* New York, Appleton-Century-Crofts, 1951.

Kraybill, William H., and Crawford, York E.: A selective medium and color test for *Mycoplasma pneumoniae. Soc Exp Biol Med, 118:*965-70, 1965.

Kubica, G.P., and Vestal, A.L.: *Tuberculosis—Laboratory Methods in Diagnosis.* Washington, D.C., U.S. Government Printing Office, 1959.

Laboratory Procedures in Clinical Bacteriology. Department of the Army, 1963.

Levinson, Samuel A., and MacFate, Robert P.: *Clinical Laboratory Diagnosis.* Philadelphia, Lea and Febiger, 1961.

Levinson, Samuel A., and MacFate, Robert P.: *Clinical Laboratory Diagnosis.* Philadelphia, Lea and Febiger, 1951.

Long, E.S.: The germ of tuberculosis, *Sci Am, 192:*1021, 1955.

Lynch, Matthew J., Raphael, Stanley S., Mellor, Leslie D., Spare, Peter D., Hills, Peter, and Inwood, Martin, J.H.: *Medical Laboratory Technology.* Philadelphia and London, W.B. Saunders, 1963.

MacFate, Robert P.: *Introduction to the Clinical Laboratory.* Chicago, Year Book Medical Publishers, 1961.

McManus, J.F.A., and Mowry, Robert W.: *Staining Methods.* New York, Paul B. Hoeber, 1960.

Miller, Seward E.: *A Textbook of Clinical Pathology.* Baltimore, Williams and Wilkins, 1960.

Needham, George Hubert: *The Practical Use of the Microscope.* Springfield, Thomas, 1958.

Neter, Erwin, and Edgeworth, D.R.: *Medical Microbiology,* 4th ed. Philadelphia, F.A. Davis, 1962.

Paine, T.F., Muray, R., Perlmutter, I., and Finland, M.: Brain abscess and meningitis associated with a pleuropneumonia-like organism: Clinical and bacteriological observations in a case with recovery. *Ann Intern Med, 32:*554, 1950.

Parsons, Rose Morgan, and Schermeister, Leo J.: An indirect hemagglutination test for *Mycoplasma pneumoniae. Am J Med Technol,* August, 1968.

Parsons, Rose Morgan, and Schermeister, Leo J.: Correlation of *Mycoplasma pneumoniae* agglutinins with the complete blood count. *Am J Med Technol,* September, 1968.

Parsons, Rose Morgan, and Schermeister, Leo J.: *The Mycoplasma.* N.D. Newsletter, 1968.

Raffel, Sidney: Basic contributions to medicine by research in microbiology. *JAMA, 179:*360, 1962.

Rosebury, T.: *Microorganisms Indigenous to Man.* New York, McGraw-Hill, 1962.

Rothenberg, Robert E.: *The New Illustrated Medical Encyclopedia for Home Use.* New York, Abradale Press Publishers, 1959, vol. 4.

Salle, A.J.: *Fundamental Principles of Bacteriology.* New York, McGraw-Hill, 1961.

Schaub, I.G., and Foley, M.K.: *Diagnostic Bacteriology,* 5th ed. St. Louis, C.V. Mosby, 1958.

Scott, E.G.: A practical blood cultures procedure. *Amer J Clin Pathol, 21:*290 1951.

Schneierson, Stanley S.: *Atlas of Diagnostic Microbiology.* North Chicago, Abbott Laboratories, 1966.

Simmons, James Stevens, and Gentzkow, Cleon J.: *Medical and Public Health Laboratory Methods.* Philadelphia, Lea and Febiger, 1956.

Simpson, W.G., and Brown, W.J.: Current status of the diagnosis and management of gonorrhea. *JAMA, 182:*63, 1962.

Slingerland, H.J., and Morgan, H.R.: Sustained bacteremia with pleuropneumonia-like organsims in post-partum patient. *JAMA, 150:*1309, 1952.

Smille, Wilson G., and Kilbourne, E.D.: *Preventive Medicine and Public Health,* New York, MacMillian, 1963.

Smith, Alice Lorraine: *Principles of Microbiology.* St. Louis, C.V. Mosby, 1965.

Smith, Alice Lorraine: *Microbiology and Pathology,* 8th ed. St. Louis, C.V. Mosby, 1964.

Smith, David T.: *Zinsser Microbiology,* 13th ed. New York, Appleton-Century-Crofts, 1964.

Smith, Edward B., Beamer, Parker, R., Vellios, Frank, and Schulz, Dale M.: *Principles of Human Pathology.* New York, Oxford University Press, 1959.

Smith, Louis D.S.: *The Pathogenic Anaerobic Bacteria*. Springfield, Thomas, 1969.

Somerson, Norman L., Walls, Barbara, and Chanock, Robert E.: Hemolysin of *Mycoplasma pneumoniae:* Tentative Identification as a peroxide. *Science, 150:369,* 1965.

Specialized Diagnostic Laboratory Tests. Bio-Science Laboratories, Los Angeles, 1961.

Stableforth, A.W., and Galloway, I.A.: *Diseases Due to Bacteria.* New York, Academic Press, 1959, Vols. I and II.

Stefanini, Mario: *Progress in Clinical Pathology.* New York and London, Grune and Stratton, 1966, Vol. I.

Stokes, E. Joan: *Clinical Bacteriology,* 3rd ed. London, Edward Arnold Publishers, 1968.

Thompson, LaVerne Ruth: *Introduction to Microorganisms.* Philadelphia, W.B. Saunders, 1954.

Tissue Culture and Virus Propagation, 4th ed. Difco Laboratories, Detroit, 1964.

Top, Franklin H.: *Communicable and Infectious Diseases.* St. Louis, C.V. Mosby, 1960.

TTC wins high praise as mass bacteriuria test. *Antibiotic News, 3:20,* 1966.

Udenfriend, Sidney: *Fluorescence Assay in Biology and Medicine.* New York, Academic Press, 1962.

Wedberg, Stanley E.: *Paramedical Microbiology.* New York, Reinhold Publishing, 1963.

Wells, Benjamin B.: *Clinical Pathology.* Philadelphia and London, W.B. Saunders, 1962.

Wells, Benjamin B.: *Clinical Pathology, Application and Interpretation,* 2nd ed. Philadelphia and London, W.B. Saunders, 1956.

Wentworth, Berttina B.: Bacteriophage typing of staphylococci. *Bacteriol Rev, 27:3,* 1963.

Wilson, G.S., and Miles, A.A.: *Topley and Wilson's Principles of Bacteriology and Immunity.* Baltimore, Williams and Wilkins, 1955, Vols. I and II.

SECTION II
MYCOLOGY

ACTINOMYCES IDENTIFICATION

SYNONYM: *Actinomyces israelii (bovis)* Identification.

NURSES' RESPONSIBILITY:

Actinomyces may appear grossly in various discharges and specimens in the form of small yellow granules ("sulfur granules"), each about the size of a pinhead. It is the responsibility of the nurse to search and report the finding of any such sulfur granules. It is also the responsibility of the nurse to assist the physician in obtaining tissue culture specimens for histopathological studies. All clinical specimens must be transported to the laboratory as soon as they have been collected.

PRINCIPLE OF THE TEST:

Actinomycosis is an infectious disease of man and animals which is caused by fungi belonging to the genus *Actinomyces*. The one of interest in man is *A. israelii (bovis)*.

Several diagnostic tests are available for diagnosing actinomycosis. Among these are the direct microscopic examination, stained smear, culture, fluorescent antibody, sugar fermentation studies, and histopathological studies.

Direct Microscopic Examination: A sulfur granule is crushed on a slide and a coverglass pressed upon it. The preparation is examined microscopically for a tangled mass of branching filaments, which is characteristic of the *Actinomyces* ("ray fungus").

Stained Smear: A Gram stain (see p. 59) may be helpful in diagnosing the *Actinomyces;* however, it must be remembered that finding of the sulfur granules and microscopic examination is *presumptive* evidence of actinomycosis. Isolation of the *A. israelii* organism from infected lesions, in addition to positive fluorescent antibody findings, provides *conclusive* evidence.

Culture: Two sets of media are inoculated; one set is incubated aerobically and one anaerobically. Aliquots of the test material are serially streaked on plates of brain-heart infusion medium containing 2% blood agar, and incubated under anaerobiosis of 5% carbon dioxide for four to six days at 37°C. After the incubation, the colonies are examined for the characteristic rough white *A. israelii* colonies. Isolation may also be accomplished by employing tubes containing glucose infusion broth under aerobic conditions and incubated at 37°C for four to six days.

Carbohydrate Fermentation Studies: Carbohydrate fermentation studies may be employed, particularly in the cases of differentiation of *A. israelii* from anaerobic *Corynebacterium* and anaerobic *Lactobacillus*. *A. israelii* produces acid and gas with maltose, xylose, salicin, levulose, raffinose, galactose, mannitol, sucrose, and dextrose; lactose is variable. The catalase test is also of use in differentiating *A. israelii* from other organisms (see *Catalase Test,* p. 30).

Histopathological Studies: Actinomyces may be demonstrated in tissues by staining with hematoxylin and eosin, as well as by MacCallum-Goodpasture bacterial stains.

SPECIMEN REQUIRED: Clinical sources include bone lesions, bronchial washings, intestinal lesions, mucosal lesions, surgical specimens, sputum, spinal fluid, draining sinuses, excised tissue, exudates, and numerous others.

PRESERVATIVE:

None is required. The material must be examined directly and cultured while fresh.

LENGTH OF TIME REQUIRED TO PERFORM TEST:

Allow a minimum of one hour for direct microscopic examination and stained smears, and up to four to six days for cultures. Fluorescent antibody tests require three to six hours for completion.

NORMAL VALUES:

No pathogenic varieties of *Actinomyces* found by laboratory identification methods. Certain varieties of the *Actinomyces* may be found in the normal mouth, pharynx, and intestine.

POSITIVE IN: Actinomycosis.

ASPERGILLUS IDENTIFICATION

SYNONYM: *Aspergillus fumigatus* Identification.

NURSES' RESPONSIBILITY:

It is the responsibility of the nurse to assist the physician in obtaining the test material and to transport it to the laboratory as soon after collection as possible.

PRINCIPLE OF THE TEST:

Aspergillosis is an acute or chronic, granulomatous infection affecting the lungs, bronchi, sinuses, and various other parts of the body. The infection is most often caused by *A. fumigatus,* although other species of *Aspergillus* may be involved.

The organism is easily identified by growth on Sabouraud's glucose agar (without acti dione) in three to five days as a grayish-blue, bluish-green, cottony colony. Macroscopically, it resembles *Penicillium;* however, the two are differentiated by direct microscopic examination. Other laboratory tests are usually not required for identification of this organism, although histopathological studies may be employed. In the latter case, the best stains are modified periodic acid-Schiff, Grocott's methenamine silver, and Gridley fungus stains. Eosin and hematoxylin are also frequently used.

SPECIMEN REQUIRED:

Clinical specimen sources include bronchial washings, sputum, surgical specimens, sinus drainings, and others.

PRESERVATIVE:

None is permitted. The material should be examined directly and cultured while fresh.

LENGTH OF TIME REQUIRED TO PERFORM TEST:

A minimum of one hour for direct microscopic examination and up to seven days for cultures should be allowed.

NORMAL VALUES: No organisms typical of *A. fumigatus* isolated.

POSITIVE IN: Aspergillosis.

BLASTOMYCES IDENTIFICATION

SYNONYM: *Blastomyces dermatitidis* Identification.

NURSES' RESPONSIBILITY:

It is the responsibility of the nurse to assist the physician in obtaining the test specimens and to transport them to the laboratory immediately after collection. Frequently, the test material will be skin scrapings, pus from an abscess, or sputum. Refer to *Sputum (Routine)*, page 86 and *Sputum Culture*, page 91 for nurses' responsibility and collection of the specimens.

PRINCIPLE OF THE TEST:

North American blastomycosis (Gilchrist's Disease) is a pulmonary, systemic, or cutaneous disease caused by *B. dermatitidis*.

Several tests are available for diagnosing North American blastomycosis. Among these are the direct microscopic examination, culture, fluorescent antibody, histopathological studies, and skin tests.

Direct Microscopic Examination: An aliquot of the test material is mounted on a slide with either a drop of 10% potassium hydroxide or sodium hydroxide; it is coverslipped and examined microscopically for the typically large, spherical, thick-walled *single-budding*, yeastlike cells, approximately 15 to 20 micra in diameter.

Culture: B. dermatitidis is difficult to culture because of secondary invaders, but may be grown on all common laboratory media. The material is cultured on blood agar or beef infusion agar at 37°C for four to ten days and is then examined for the characteristic growth. Sabouraud's glucose agar (containing antibiotics) may also be used, in which case the culture is grown at room temperature and thereafter examined at four to ten days for characteristic growth.

Histopathological Studies: B. dermatitidis may be demonstrated in tissues stained with hematoxylin and eosin, or by Grocott's methenamine silver and modified periodic acid-Schiff stains.

Skin Tests: Because of cross-immunity between histoplasmosis and blastomycosis, the patient must be tested with both antigens simultaneously.

SPECIMEN REQUIRED:

Clinical specimen sources include abscesses, sputum, liver, spleen, prostate gland, kidneys, pleural exudates, bone lesions, bronchial washings, cutaneous lesions, lymph nodes, spinal fluid, surgical specimens, and urine.

PRESERVATIVE:

None is permitted. The material must be examined directly and cultured while fresh.

LENGTH OF TIME REQUIRED TO PERFORM TEST:

A minimum of one hour for direct microscopic examination and up to several weeks for cultures should be allowed.

NORMAL VALUES:

No organisms characteristic of *B. dermatitidis* found by laboratory identification methods.

POSITIVE IN: North American blastomycosis.

CANDIDA IDENTIFICATION

SYNONYM: *Candida albicans* Identification.

NURSES' RESPONSIBILITY:

It is the responsibility of the nurse to assist the physician in obtaining the test specimens and to transport them to the laboratory immediately after the collection. Frequently, blood, spinal fluid, or sputum will be the material of choice.

PRINCIPLE OF THE TEST:

Candidiasis is a localized or generalized disease caused by *C. albicans* (and other species of *Candida*).

Several tests are available for diagnosing candidiasis. Among these are the direct microscopic examination, stained smear, culture, fluorescent antibody, histopathological studies, and a few other tests.

Direct Microscopic Examination: An aliquot of the skin scrapings is mounted on a slide with either 10% potassium hydroxide or sodium hydroxide; it is heated, coverslipped, and examined for the characteristic small, oval, budding or nonbudding yeast cells, about three to six micra in diameter. Sputum, vaginal materials, and a few others should be mixed in saline, coverslipped, and examined microscopically (see *TYN Test,* p. 101).

Stained Smear: An aliquot of the test material is placed on a slide, allowed to air-dry, fixed by flame, and stained by Gram's method (see p. 59). The preparation is then examined microscopically for the characteristic morphology.

Culture: The test material is cultured on Sabouraud glucose agar (with antibiotics) and incubated at 37°C and at room temperature, and examined at one to four days for characteristic growth.

Histopathological Studies: C. albicans may be demonstrated in tissues readily with Grocott's methenamine silver technique, modified periodic acid-Schiff, and Gram stains.

Other Tests: Carbohydrate fermentation studies may be helpful in the identification of *C. albicans*. Acid and gas are formed in glucose and maltose, whereas only acid is formed in sucrose.

No acid or gas is formed in lactose. Animal inoculation may also be helpful in some cases (refer to *Animal Inoculation,* p. 9).

SPECIMEN REQUIRED:

Clinical specimens such as blood, bronchial washings, abscesses, cutaneous lesions, mucosal lesions, spinal fluid, sputum, stools, surgical specimens, and urine may be used.

PRESERVATIVE:

None is permitted. The material must be examined directly and cultured while fresh.

LENGTH OF TIME REQUIRED TO PERFORM TEST:

A minimum of one hour for direct microscopic examination and up to seven days for cultures should be allowed.

NORMAL VALUES:

No pathogenic strains of *C. albicans* found in superficial infections.

POSITIVE IN: Candidiasis.

COCCIDIOIDES IDENTIFICATION

SYNONYM: *Coccidioides immitis* Identification.

NURSES' RESPONSIBILITY:

It is the responsibility of the nurse to assist the physician in obtaining the test specimens and to transport these to the laboratory immediately after collection. *Great care must be exercised in the handling of test materials since the arthrospores are highly infectious and may be easily dispersed when moved.*

PRINCIPLE OF THE TEST:

Coccidioides is an acute, highly infectious, dust-borne, benign respiratory disease caused by *C. immitis.*

Several diagnostic tests are available for diagnosing coccidioidosis. Among these are the direct microscopic examination, culture, fluorescent antibody, histopathological studies, and skin tests.

Direct Microscopic Examination: An aliquot of the test material is mounted on a slide with one drop either 10% potassium hydroxide or sodium hydroxide; it is coverslipped and examined for the typical, thick-walled spherules, 15 to 80 micra in diameter, and containing numerous small endospores, two to five micra in diameter.

Culture: C. immitis can be grown at room temperature on all common laboratory media. The material is usually cultured on Sabouraud's glucose agar (containing antibiotics) at room temperature for four to six days and then examined for the characteristic growth.

Histopathological Studies: C. immitis may be demonstrated in tissues stained with hematoxylin and eosin, or by Grocott's methenamine silver stain.

SPECIMEN REQUIRED:

Clinical specimen sources include abscesses, sputum, pleural fluid, exudates, gastric contents, bone lesions, cutaneous lesions, surgical specimens, feces, and urine.

PRESERVATIVE:

None is permitted. The material should be examined directly and cultured while fresh.

LENGTH OF TIME REQUIRED TO PERFORM TEST:

A minimum of one hour for direct microscopic examination and up to several weeks for culture should be allowed.

NORMAL VALUES:

No organisms typical of *C. immitis* found by laboratory identification methods.

POSITIVE IN: Coccidioidomycosis.

CRYPTOCOCCUS IDENTIFICATION

SYNONYMS: *Cryptococcus neoformans* Identification; *Torula histo-lytica* Identification.

NURSES' RESPONSIBILITY:

It is the responsibility of the nurse to assist the physician in the collection of the test materials and to transport these to the laboratory immediately after the collection.

PRINCIPLE OF THE TEST:

Cryptococcosis is an infectious disease caused by the patho-genic yeast, *C. neoformans (Torula histolytica)*.

Several diagnostic tests are available for diagnosing crypto-coccosis. Among these are the direct microscopic examination, culture, fluorescent antibody, and histopathological studies.

Direct Microscopic Examination: The test material is mounted on a slide with one drop either of 10% potassium hydroxide or sodium hydroxide; it is coverslipped and examined microscopic-ally. The preparation is often stained with Mayer's mucicarmine stain, which is specific for *C. neoformans,* since it selectively stains the mucinous capsule. If "grains" and "granules" are observed, they are crushed and Gram stained (see Gram stain, p. 59). If any budding cells are found, a drop of 50% India ink is added as a mount to check the cells for capsules. *C. neoformans* appears as thick-walled, oval, budding, encapsulated yeast cells, five to twenty micra in diameter.

Culture: C neoformans may be cultured on most laboratory media. The material is cultured on blood agar or Sabouraud's glucose agar at room temperature and at 35°C for four to seven days. Virulent species of *C. neoformans* grow at 35°C, while the nonvirulent species do not. Identification may be verified by microscopic examination.

Histopathological Studies: C. neoformans may be demon-strated in tissues by staining with hematoxylin and eosin but even more readily by employing modified periodic acid-Schiff, Gram stain (see p. 59), Gridley fungus stain, or Grocott's methenamine silver method. The preparation may also be stained with Mayer's mucicarmine stain which is specific for *C. neoformans* since it selectively stains the mucinous capsule.

SPECIMEN REQUIRED:

Clinical specimen materials include sources such as bone lesions, bronchial washings, cutaneous lesions, abscesses, draining sinus tracts, lymph nodes, mucosal lesions, spinal fluid, sputum, surgical specimens, urine, and others.

PRESERVATIVE:

None is permitted. The material should be examined directly and cultured while fresh.

LENGTH OF TIME REQUIRED TO PERFORM TEST:

A minimum of one hour for direct microscopic examination and up to four to six days for cultures should be allowed.

NORMAL VALUES:

No organisms typical of *C. neoformans* found by laboratory identification methods.

POSITIVE IN: Cryptococcosis.

EPIDERMOPHYTON IDENTIFICATION

SYNONYM: *Epidermophyton floccosum* Identification.

NURSES' RESPONSIBILITY:

It is the responsibility of the nurse to assist the physician in obtaining the test specimens and to transport these to the laboratory immediately after collection.

PRINCIPLE OF THE TEST:

The genus *Epidermophyton* contains one species of importance to man, *E. floccosum*, which invades the skin and nails, but *not* the hair.

Laboratory tests for the identification of *E. floccosum* include the direct microscopic examination, culture, and fluorescent antibody.

Direct Microscopic Examination: A few finely chopped nails or skin scrapings are mounted on a glass slide in a drop of 10% potassium hydroxide or sodium hydroxide; they are coverglassed, heated, and examined microscopically for characteristic morphology, which is identified by broadly clavate (club-shaped), two- to six-celled, smooth, thin-walled macroconidia. No microconidia are present.

Culture: E. floccosum is most often cultured on Sabouraud's glucose agar (containing antibiotics) at room temperature for four to six days and then examined for characteristic growth of greenish-yellow, velvety to powdery, rapidly growing colonies.

SPECIMEN REQUIRED:

A few skin scrapings or nail clippings are required.

PRESERVATIVE: None is permitted.

LENGTH OF TIME REQUIRED TO PERFORM TEST:

Allow a minimum of one hour for direct microscopic examination and up to 10 days for cultures.

NORMAL VALUES:

No organisms characteristic of *E. floccosum* identified by laboratory methods.

POSITIVE IN: Athlete's foot, tinea cruris.

FUNGUS IDENTIFICATION (GENERAL METHODS)

Medically important fungi are divided into three broad classes, depending on the disease produced. The largest group is that of the *systemic mycoses* (deep mycoses), which includes actinomycosis, aspergillosis, blastomycosis (North and South American), candidiasis, coccidioidomycosis, cryptococcosis, histoplasmosis, and nocardiosis. The *superficial mycoses* (dermatophytes) include the *Trichophyton, Epidermophyton,* and *Microsporum,* while the *intermediate mycoses* include candidiasis (sometimes), chromomycosis, and sporotrichosis. The intermediate mycoses may include some of the superficial group and may develop into systemic mycoses.

Various diagnostic methods are currently being employed in the identification of fungi of medical importance. Among the more frequently requested are the direct microscopic examination, stained smear, culture, fluorescent antibody, skin tests, histopathological studies, serological tests, and animal inoculation. Each of these methods is briefly described here, and the reader is referred to the individual fungus identification tests included in this section.

Direct Microscopic Examination: A small drop of the test material is mounted on a chemically clean glass slide with a drop of either 10% potassium hydroxide or sodium hydroxide to dissolve extraneous materials such as debris; the slide is coverslipped and examined microscopically for the typical cells.

Stained Smear: A drop of the test material is placed on a chemically clean slide, smeared, allowed to air-dry, and stained by a dye such as Giemsa's or Wright's. The preparation is coverslipped and examined microscopically for the characteristic cells.

Culture: Various fungi require different laboratory media for growth. However, most fungi grow well on blood agar, brain-heart infusion agar, and Sabouraud's glucose agar. Other media, such as Littman's medium, Mycosel broth/agar, and eosin methylene blue (EMB), may be used. Certain cultures of organisms, such as those of the *Actinomyces,* may require anaerobic growth with 5% carbon dioxide or 95% nitrogen. Various cultures which are negative may be held and examined at intervals for three to four weeks before being reported as negative. Frequently, two sets of media are inoculated with the test organism; one is incubated at room temperature (22° to 25°C) and the other at 35° to 37°C.

Fluorescent Antibody: Diagnosis may frequently be accelerated by use of the fluorescent antibody in direct tissue preparation. Refer to the section on *Fluorescent Antibody,* page 52, for a detailed description of the procedure.

Skin Tests: Skin tests may be of value in conjunction with other laboratory tests in the identification of fungal diseases.

Histopathological Studies: Tissue sectioning is of extreme value in the diagnosis of various systemic fungi.

Serologic Tests: Tests for complement-fixing antibodies, hemagglutinins, agglutinins, and precipitins are available for several organisms, such as *Coccidioides immitis, Histoplasma capsulatum,* and *Blastomyces dermatitidis.* Generally speaking, these are considered unsatisfactory for diagnostic use due to cross-reactions.

Animal Inoculation: Animal inoculation may be required in some cases of fungi identification when time is not of the essence and other laboratory tests prove nonfruitful in diagnosis. Refer to *Animal Inoculation,* page 9, for a complete description.

Other Tests: Occasionally, other tests may be requested in conjunction with the more frequently used methods listed above. These might include carbohydrate fermentation tests, catalase tests, and other biochemical tests.

FUNGI — NOMENCLATURE

Certain fungi are known to clinicians by various terminology. The following is a listing of the preferred names of the various fungi, as well as some of the most commonly known synonyms.

FUNGI—PREFERRED NAMES AND SYNONYMS

PREFERRED NAME	SYNONYM(S):
Absidia corymbifera	*Mucor corymbifer.*
Aspergillus fumigatus	*A. bronchialis.*
Blastomyces brasiliensis	*Paracoccidioides brasiliensis.*
Blastomyces dermatitidis	*Zymonema dermatitidis.*
Candida albicans	*Monilia albicans, Oidium albicans.*
Cladosporium mansoni	*Torula mansoni.*
Cryptococcus neoformans	*C. meningitidis, Torula histolytica, Torulopsis neoformans.*
Epidermophyton floccosum	*E. clypeiforme, E. cruris, E. inguinale, Trichophyton cruris, T. intertriginis.*
Histoplasma capsulatum	*Cryptococcus capsulatus.*
Hormodendron pedrosoi	*Fonsecaea pedrosoi, Phialophora pedrosoi.*
Hormodendron verrucosa	*Cadophora americana, Phialophora verrucosa.*
Malassezia furfur	*Microsporum furfur.*
Microsporum audouini	*Sabouraudites audouini, Trichophyton declavans.*
Microsporum gypseum	*Achorion gypseum, M. fulvum, Sabouraudites gypseus.*
Monosporium apiospermum	*Allescheria boydii, Glenospora boydii, Indiella americana.*
Trichophyton flavum	*T. cerebriforme, T. epilans.*
Trichophyton interdigitale	*Ctenomyces interdigitalis, Epidermophyton interdigitale.*
Trichophyton mentagrophytes	*Ctenomyces asteroides, C. mentagrophytes, T. asteroides, T. gypseum.*
Trichophyton rubrum	*Epidermophyton rubrum, T. purpureum.*

131

Trichophyton schoenleini	*Achorion schoenleini,* *Oidium schoenleini.*
Trichophyton tonsurans	*T. crateriforme.*
Trichophyton violaceum	*Achorion violaceum.*

FUNGI—SPECIMENS AND PRINCIPLE
ETIOLOGIC AGENTS

SITE OF INFECTION	CLINICAL SPECIMENS	PRINCIPLE ETIOLOGIC AGENTS
Abscess	Purulent material from lesion.	Actinomyces spp., *Blastomyces brasiliensis*, *Blastomyces dermatitidis*, *Candida albicans*, *Coccidioides immitis*, *Cryptococcus neoformans*, *Histoplasma capsulatum*, *Hormodendrum pedrosoi*, *Monosporium apiospermum*, *Nocardia asteroides*, *Sporotrichum schenckii*.
Aorta	Purulent material from lesion.	*Blastomyces brasiliensis*, *Blastomyces dermatitidis*, *Cryptococcus neoformans*.
Blood	5 ml of venous blood anticoagulated with heparin.	*Blastomyces brasiliensis*, *Blastomyces dermatitidis*, *Candida albicans*, *Histoplasma capsulatum*, *Nocardia asteroides*.
Bone Marrow	0.2 to 0.5 ml of bone marrow, anticoagulated with EDTA or heparin.	*Actinomyces israelii*, *Blastomyces brasiliensis*, *Blastomyces dermatitidis*, *Coccidioides immitis*, *Cryptococcus neoformans*, *Histoplasma capsulatum*, *Microsporum apiospermum* (foot only), *Nocardia asteroides*, *Sporotrichum schenckii*.
Cerebrospinal Fluid	4.0 to 5.0 ml of fresh spinal fluid.	*Actinomyces israelii*, *Blastomyces dermatitidis*, *Blastomyces brasiliensis*,

133

		Candida albicans, *Coccidioides immitis,* *Cryptococcus neoformans,* *Histoplasma capsulatum,* *Nocardia asteroides.*
Ear (External)	Few scrapings from external ear, or two sterile swabs from drainage in Mycosel tubes.	*Blastomyces brasiliensis,* *Blastomyces dermatitidis,* *Candida albicans,* *Coccidioides immitis,* *Cryptococcus neoformans,* *Epidermophyton.* *Histoplasma capsulatum,* *Hormodendrum pedrosoi,* *Microsporum,* *Nocardia asteroides,* *Sporotrichum schenckii,* *Trichophyton.*
Eye	A few drops of fluid from the lacrimal duct or eye scrapings in sterile saline or Sabouraud's broth.	*Sporotrichum schenckii.*
Feces	A few grams of fecal material.	*Blastomyces brasiliensis,* *Candida albicans,* *Coccidioides immitis,* *Geotrichum candidum.*
Gastric Lavage	8 to 10 ml of gastric washings.	*Blastomyces brasiliensis,* *Blastomyces dermatitidis.*
Hair	16 to 20 hairs put into a clean, white envelope or placed on glass slides, sterile test tubes, or petridishes.	*Epidermophyton,* *Microsporum,* *Trichophyton.*
Larynx	Purulent material from lesion.	*Blastomyces brasiliensis,* *Blastomyces dermatitidis,* *Coccidioides immitis,* *Cryptococcus neoformans,* *Histoplasma capsulatum.*

Liver	Biopsy obtained by needle puncture or surgical removal.	*Blastomyces brasiliensis, Blastomyces dermatitidis, Candida albicans, Cryptococcus neoformans, Histoplasma capsulatum, Nocardia asteroides.*
Lymph Nodes	Biopsy obtained by surgical technique.	*Blastomyces brasiliensis, Blastomyces dermatitidis, Candida albicans, Cryptococcus neoformans, Histoplasma capsulatum, Nocardia asteroides, Sporotrichum schenckii.*
Mouth Scrapings	A few scrapings obtained from the oral cavity, in sterile saline.	*Blastomyces brasiliensis, Candida albicans, Histoplasma capsulatum.*
Nails: Toe—Finger	Portion of the nail, the entire nail, or exudate from the nail in a sterile test tube or petri dish.	*Candida albicans, Epiderophyton, Microsporum, Trichophyton.*
Pancreas	Biopsy obtained by surgical technique.	*Cryptococcus neoformans, Histoplasma capsulatum, Nocardia asteroides.*
Penile Lesion	Impression smear of the exudate or tube of Mycosel broth.	*Blastomyces brasiliensis, Blastomyces dermatitidis, Candida albicans, Coccidioides immitis, Cryptococcus neoformans, Epidermophyton, Histoplasma capsulatum, Hormodendrum pedrosoi, Microsporum, Nocardia asteroides, Sporotrichum schenckii, Trichophyton.*

Pharynx	Purulent material from lesion.	*Histoplasma capsulatum, Nocardia asteroides.*
Prostate	Material obtained from prostatic massage or by surgery.	*Blastomyces dermatitidis, Nocardia asteroides.*
Skin	A few skin scrapings from periphery of the lesion put in a sterile petri dish or between two flamed glass slides.	*Blastomyces brasiliensis, Blastomyces dermatitidis, Candida albicans, Coccidioides immitis, Cryptococcus neoformans, Epidermophyton, Histoplasma capsulatum, Hormodendrum pedrosoi, Monosporium apiospermum* (Foot only) *Microsporum, Nocardia asteroides, Sporotrichum schenckii, Trichophyton.*
Spleen	Biopsy obtained by needle puncture or surgical removal.	*Blastomyces brasiliensis, Blastomyces dermatitidis, Candida albicans, Cryptococcus neoformans, Histoplasma capsulatum, Nocardia asteroides.*
Sputum	Fresh sputum obtained in the early morning and placed in a sterile petri dish.	*Actinomyces israelii, Aspergillus fumigatus, Blastomyces brasiliensis, Blastomyces dermatitidis, Candida albicans, Coccidioides immitis, Cryptococcus neoformans, Geotrichum candidum, Histoplasma capsulatum, Nocardia asteroides, Sporotrichum schenckii.*

Thyroid	Purulent material from lesion.	*Cryptococcus neoformans, Histoplasma capsulatum.*
Ulcer	A small sterile gauze square containing the lesion, in a sterile petri dish.	*Blastomyces brasiliensis, Blastomyces dermatitidis, Candida albicans, Coccidioides immitis, Cryptococcus neoformans, Epidermophyton, Histoplasma capsulatum, Hormodendrum pedrosoi, Microsporum, Nocardia asteroides, Sporotrichum schenckii, Trichophyton.*
Urine	2 to 5 ml of a catheterized or "clean-catch" specimen in a sterile tube or bottle.	*Blastomyces dermatitidis, Candida albicans, Coccidioides immitis, Cryptococcus neoformans, Histoplasma capsulatum.*
Vaginal Material	A few milliliters of a vaginal-saline washing in a sterile test tube.	*Candida albicans.*

HISTOPLASMA IDENTIFICATION

SYNONYM: *Histoplasma capsulatum* Identification.

NURSES' RESPONSIBILITY:

It is the responsibility of the nurse to assist the physician in obtaining the test materials and to transport these to the laboratory immediately after collection. *Extreme caution* must be exercised in the handling of materials thought to be infected with *H. capsulatum,* since spores are capable of producing highly infectious aerosols.

PRINCIPLE OF THE TEST:

Histoplasmosis is an infectious disease, caused by *H. capsulatum;* it may be acute, subacute, localized, or disseminated, and it affects primarily the reticuloendothelial system.

Several diagnostic tests are necessary for positive findings of histoplasmosis. Among these are the direct stained smear, culture, fluorescent antibody, skin tests, and histopathological studies.

Direct Stained Smear: Material from the infected area is examined microscopically in an attempt to diagnose *H. capsulatum* fungus infection (histoplasmosis). An aliquot of the test material is placed on a slide, smeared, and stained with a special stain, such as Wright's, Giemsa's, or periodic acid-Schiff; it is then coverslipped and examined under the microscope for the characteristic *H. capsulatum* organisms. These appear as small, round, budding cells, approximately one to five micra in diameter, with a clear area surrounding each, somewhat like a halo. Peripheral blood smears and stained bone marrow smears should be examined and stained for the characteristic bodies in polymorphonuclear and mononuclear cells.

Culture: H. capsulatum may be cultured on most common laboratory media. An aliquot of the test material is inoculated on a blood agar slant, sealed, and incubated at 37°C. Macroscopically, these colonies appear smooth, white- to cream-colored, and yeast like; microscopically, they are the typical small, round, budding cells. Sabouraud's glucose agar (with antibiotics or cycloheximide) may also be used, in which case the culture is grown at room temperature and examined for a white- to buff-colored, cottony growth.

Skin Tests: The *Histoplasmin Skin Test* is used in the diagnosis of hisptoplasmosis; due to cross immunity it must accompanied by the blastomycin and coccidioidin skin tests.

Histopathological Studies: H. capsulatum may be demonstrated in tissues by use of the modified acid-Schiff and Grocott's methenamine silver stains. Hematoxylin and eosin may also be used.

SPECIMEN REQUIRED:

The most likely clinical specimens are blood, bone marrow, bronchial washings, cutaneous lesions, abscesses, draining sinus tracts, intestinal lesions, lymph nodes, mucosal lesions, spinal fluid, sputum, surgical specimens, and urine.

PRESERVATIVE:

None is permitted. The material should be examined directly and cultured while fresh.

LENGTH OF TIME REQUIRED TO PERFORM TEST:

A minimum of one hour for the direct smear and up to several weeks for the culture should be allowed.

NORMAL VALUES:

No organisms characteristic of *H. capsulatum* identified by laboratory identification methods.

POSITIVE IN: Histoplasmosis.

MICROSPORUM IDENTIFICATION

SYNONYMS: *Microsporum audouini* Identification, *Microsporum canis* Identification, *Microsporum gypseum* Identification.

NURSES' RESPONSIBILITY:

It is the responsibility of the nurse to assist the physician in obtaining the test specimens and to transport these to the laboratory immediately after the collection.

PRINCIPLE OF THE TEST:

The genus *Microsporum* contains three species which invade the skin and hair but rarely the nails: *M. audouini, M. canis,* and *M. gypseum.*

Laboratory identification tests for *Microsporum* include the direct microscopic examination, culture, and fluorescent antibody.

Direct Microscopic Examination: A few hairs or finely chopped nails are mounted on a glass slide and a drop of 10% potassium hydroxide or sodium hydroxide added; the slide is coverglassed, heated, and examined microscopically for characteristic morphology.

Culture: Microsporum is cultured on Sabouraud's glucose agar (containing antibiotics) at room temperature for four to seven days and then examined for characteristic growth which ranges from slow-growing and furrowed to fast-growing, powdery, tan-brown colonies. The species is determined by culture, depending on time of growth of colony, gross morphology, color and pigmentation, microscopic morphology, and other characteristics.

SPECIMEN REQUIRED:

A few hairs or finely chopped nails are needed.

PRESERVATIVE: None is permitted.

LENGTH OF TIME REQUIRED TO PERFORM TEST:

Allow one to two hours for direct examination and four to seven days for cultures.

NORMAL VALUES:

No *Microsporum* organisms identified by laboratory methods.

POSITIVE IN:

M. canis (M. lanosum): Sporadic infections in humans of ringworm of scalp and globrous skin. *M. audouini:* epidemics of tinea capitis. *M. gypseum:* Favus; infections of animals and man.

NOCARDIA IDENTIFICATION

SYNONYM: *Nocardia asteroides* Identification.

NURSES' RESPONSIBILITY:

It is the responsibility of the nurse to assist the physician in the collection of test materials and to transport these to the laboratory as soon as possible after the collection. Aseptic technique must be exercised at all times in obtaining the specimens. A careful search should be made for "granules" and reported as "granules present."

PRINCIPLE OF THE TEST:

Nocardiosis is a pulmonary, systemic disease caused by the acid-fast species, *N. asteroides,* as well as by a few other nonacid-fast *Nocardia* species.

Several diagnostic tests are available for diagnosing nocardiosis. Among these are the direct microscopic examination, stained smear, acid-fast stain (Ziehl-Neelson method), culture, fluorescent antibody, and histopathological studies.

Direct Microscopic Examination: Exudates, pus, or skin scrapings are placed on a slide, are coverglassed, and examined for characteristic *Nocardia* morphology.

Direct Stained Smear: An aliquot of the test material is placed on a glass slide and stained by Gram's method (p. 59); it is then coverslipped and examined microscopically for the typical morphology.

Acid-Fast Stain: An aliquot of the test material is placed on a glass slide, stained by the Ziehl-Neelson method (see p. 7), and examined microscopically for the typical acid-fast organisms.

Culture: All *Nocardia* species are aerobic and may be cultured on common laboratory media. The material is cultured on blood agar, which is incubated at 37°C and on Sabouraud's glucose agar, incubated at room temperature. The cultures are incubated under aerobic conditions, in contrast to *Actinomyces israelii* which is grown under anaerobic conditions.

Histopathological Studies: Nocardia may be demonstrated in tissues by staining with Grocott's methenamine silver stain. At times, the Brown and Brenn bacterial stain may be used to distinguish *Nocardia* from fibrin. Fibrin is gram-negative, while Nocardia is gram-positive. Morphologically, *Nocardia* and *Streptomyces* are indistinguishable.

SPECIMEN REQUIRED:

Clinical specimen sources include bone lesions, cutaneous lesions, abscesses, draining sinus tracts, surgical specimens, sputum, or exudates.

PRESERVATIVE:

None is permitted. The material should be examined directly and cultured while fresh.

LENGTH OF TIME REQUIRED TO PERFORM TEST:

Allow a minimum of one hour for direct and stained smears and four to six days for cultures.

NORMAL VALUES:

No organisms typical of *N. asteroides* found by laboratory identification methods.

POSITIVE IN: Nocardiosis.

PARACOCCIDIOIDES IDENTIFICATION

SYNONYMS: *Paracoccidioides brasiliensis* Identification, *Blastomyces brasiliensis* Identification.

NURSES' RESPONSIBILITY:

It is the responsibility of the nurse to assist the physician in obtaining the test specimens and to transport them to the laboratory as soon as possible after collection.

PRINCIPLE OF THE TEST:

South American blastomycosis is a chronic cutaneous, visceral, or lymphangitic disease which may occur in mixed form. It is very similar to North American blastomycosis.

Several diagnostic tests are available for diagnosing South American blastomycosis. Among these are the direct microscopic examination, culture, fluorescent antibody, and histopathological studies.

Direct Microscopic Examination: An aliquot of the test material is mounted on a slide with either 10% potassium hydroxide or sodium hydroxide; it is coverslipped and examined microscopically for the typical large, spherical, thick-walled, *multiple-budding,* yeast-like cells approximately 10 to 60 micra in diameter.

Culture: B. brasiliensis, like *B. dermatitidis,* is difficult to culture because of secondary invaders but may be grown on most laboratory media at 37°C. The material is cultured in a like manner to *B. dermatitidis* on blood agar, chocolate blood agar, and beef infusion agar at 37°C and at room temperature for four to ten days and is then examined for the characteristic growth. If Sabouraud's glucose agar is used, antibiotics are often added; the culture is grown at room temperature and examined at four to ten days for characteristic growth.

Histopathological Studies: B. brasiliensis may be demonstrated in tissues stained with hematoxylin and eosin, or by Grocott's methenamine silver stain.

Skin Tests: Because of cross immunity between blastomycosis and histoplasmosis, the patient must be tested with both antigens simultaneously.

SPECIMEN REQUIRED:

Clinical specimen sources include abscesses, bone lesions, bronchial washings, cutaneous lesions, draining sinus tracts, intestinal lesions, lymphatics, lymph nodes, mucosal lesions, sputum, surgical specimens, and exudates.

PRESERVATIVE:

None is permitted. The material should be examined directly and cultured while fresh.

LENGTH OF TIME REQUIRED TO PERFORM TEST:

A minimum of one hour for direct microscopic examination and up to several weeks for cultures should be allowed.

NORMAL VALUES:

No organisms typical of *B. brasiliensis* found by laboratory identification methods.

POSITIVE IN: South American blastomycosis.

SUPERFICIAL MYCOSES (DERMATOPHYTES) IDENTIFICATION

The superficial mycoses (dermatophytes) are a group of closely related fungi which invade only the superficial keratinized areas of the body, such as the skin, hair, and nails. They rarely invade the subcutaneous tissues or cause systemic infections. Three genera are of medical importance, and the reader is referred to the individual identification procedures listed as

Epidermophyton Identification.

Microsporum Identification.

Trichophyton Identification.

Occasionally, *Candida* is included (see p. 122 for a description). The three genera are differentiated by the number of macroconidia produced and the presence or absence of microconidia, and they are also classified according to the area of the body involved.

146

SYSTEMIC MYCOSES IDENTIFICATION

The systemic (deep) mycoses are relatively a rare group of fungi which invade the deep areas of the body, producing severe and spreading lesions. Most often, these organisms are not transmitted from one individual to another.

The reader is referred to the individual identification procedures of the systemic mycoses, which are listed as follows:

Actinomyces Identification.
Aspergillus Identification.
Blastomyces Identification.
Candida Identification.
Coccidioides Identification.
Cryptococcus Identification.
Histoplasma Identification.
Nocardia Identification.
Paracoccidioides Identification.

SYSTEMIC MYCOSES—SYNONYMS AND ETIOLOGICAL AGENTS

DISEASE	SYNONYMS	ETIOLOGICAL AGENTS
Actinomycosis		*Actinomyces israelii (bovis).*
Aspergillosis		*Aspergillus fumigatus, A. amotelodami, A. oryzae, A. sydowi.*
Blastomycosis— North American	Gilchrist's disease	*Blastomyces dermatitidis.*
Blastomycosis— South American	Refer to *Paracoccidioidomycosis*	
Candidiasis	Moniliasis	*Candida albicans, C. tropicalis, C. guilliermondi.*
Coccidioidomycosis	Coccidioidal granuloma, Valley fever.	*Coccidioides immitis.*

147

Cryptococcosis	Busse-Buschke's disease, European blastomycosis, torulosis, *Torula* meningitis.	*Cryptococcus neoformans, (Torula histolytica).*
Histoplasmosis	Darling's Disease, reticuloendothelial cytomycosis.	*Histoplasma capsulatum.*
Nocardiosis		*Nocardia asteroides.*
Paracoccidio-mycosis	Blastomycosis—South American, Lutz—Splendore—Almeida's Disease, paracoccidiodal granuloma.	*Paracoccidioides brasiliensis (Blastomyces brasiliensis).*

TRICHOPHYTON IDENTIFICATION

Synonym: *Trichophyton* Species Identification.

Nurses' Responsibility:

It is the responsibility of the nurse to assist the physician in obtaining the test specimens and to transport these to the laboratory as soon as possible after the collection.

Principle of the Test:

The genus *Trichophyton* contains six species of interest which invade the feet, nails, and hair: *T. mentagrophytes (gypseum), T. rubrum (purpureum), T. tonsurans (crateriforme), T. schoenleini (achorion), T. violaceum (achorion),* and *T. concentricum (endodermophyton).*

In some species, spores may be lacking in some forms, and therefore direct microscopic examination is of little value. Colonial growth is identified by cultural methods. The *Trichophytin Skin Test* is of some value. Fluorescent antibody studies are also of value and are increasing in importance.

Culture: Trichophyton is cultured on Sabouraud's glucose agar (containing antibiotics) at room temperature for five to ten days. It is then examined for characteristic growth which ranges from granular to powdery, wrinkled to folded with a velvety surface to a smooth and waxy surface; cottony to velvety, pink to reddish-purple to buff. The species is determined by culture, depending on time of the growth of the colony, gross morphology of the colony, color and pigmentation, microscopic morphology, and other characteristics.

Specimen Required:

A few hairs, skin scrapings, or nail clippings are needed.

Preservative: None is permitted.

Length of Time Required to Perform Test:

Allow five to ten days for cultures.

Normal Values:

No *Trichophyton* organisms identified by laboratory methods.

POSITIVE IN:

T. mentagrophytes: Ectothrix infections of the hair and infections of the skin, beard, and nails; "athletes foot;" ringworm. *T. rubrum:* Recalcitrant lesions of skin and nails. *T. tonsurans:* Tinea capitis. *T. schoenleini:* Favus; oncychomycosis. T. *violaceum:* Ringworm; sycosis. *T. concentricum:* Tinea imbricate (Tokelau).

REFERENCES

Anderson, W.A.D.: *Pathology*, 5th ed. St. Louis, C.V. Mosby, 1966.

Aravysky, A.N.: Rare mycological findings in pathological material. *Mycopathologia, 16:*177-193, 1962.

Bacon, A.E., Jr., Scott, E.G., and Huntington, P.W.: Meningoencephalitis due to *Cryptococcus neoformans (Torula histolytica). Del Med J,* pp. 3-8, 1954.

Bailey, W., and Scott, Elvyn G.: Diagnostic Microbiology, 2nd ed. St. Louis, C.V. Mosby, 1966.

Bailey, W., and Scott, Elvyn G.: Diagnostic Microbiology, St. Louis, C.V. Mosby, 1962.

Barter, A.P., and Falconer, M.A.: Actinomycosis of the brain: Report of a successfully treated case. *Guys Hosp Rep, 104:*35-45, 1955.

Bauer, John D., Toro, Gelson, and Ackermann, Philip G.: *Bray's Clinical Laboratory Methods.* St. Louis, C.V. Mosby, 1962.

Beneke, E.S.: *Medical Mycology—Laboratory Manual.* Minneapolis, Burgess Publishing, 1957.

Benham, R.W.: Cryptococci—Their identification by morphology and serology. *J Infect Dis, 57:*255-274, 1935.

Boshes, L.D., Sherman, I.C., Hesser, C.J., Milzer, A., and MacLean, H.: Fungus infections of the central nervous system: Experience in treatment of cryptococcosis with cycloheximide (actidione). *Arch Neurol Psychiatr, 75:*175-197, 1956.

Boyd, William: *An Introduction to the Study of Medicine,* 5th ed. Philadelphia, Lea and Febiger, 1961.

Breed, Robert S., Murray, E.G.D., and Smith, Nathan R.: *Bergey's Manual of Determinative Bacteriology, 7th ed.* Baltimore, Williams and Wilkins, 1957.

Brine, J.A.: Human nocardiosis—A developing clinical picture. *Med J Aust, 1:*339-342, 1965.

Bunnel, I.L.: A report of ten proved cases of histoplasmosis. *Public Health Rep, 63:*299-316, 1948.

Burrows, William: *Textbook of Microbiology,* 18th ed. Philadelphia and London, W.B. Saunders, 1963.

Burrows, William: *Textbook of Microbiology,* 17th ed. Philadelphia and London, W.B. Saunders, 1959.

Buss, W.C., Gibson, T.E., and Gifford, M.A.: Coccidioidomycosis of meninges. *Calif Med, 72:*167-169, 1950.

Butler, W.T., Alling, D.W., Spickard, A., and Utz, J.P.: Diagnostic and prognostic value of clinical and laboratory findings in cryptococcal meningitis: A follow-up study of forty patients. *N Eng J Med, 270:*59-67, 1964.

Callaway, J.L., and Martin, Donald: *Manual of Clinical Mycology,* 2nd ed. Philadelphia, W.B. Saunders Co., 1954.

Canton, C.A., and Liebig, C.S.: Treatment of central nervous system cryptococcosis: Laboratory studies. *Arch Intern Med, 91:*773-783, 1953.

Chapnick, H.A.: Disseminated coccidioidomyocsis. *J Mich Med Soc, 51:*833-836, 1952.

Cherniss, E.I., and Waisbren, B.A.: North American blastomycosis; A clinical study of 40 cases. *Ann Intern Med, 44:*105-123, 1956.

Cooper, R.A., and Goldstein, E.: Histoplasmosis of the central nervous system: A report of two cases and review of literature. *Am J Med, 35:* 45-57, 1963.

Damm, Henry C.: *Practical Manual for Clinical Laboratory Procedures.* Cleveland, Chemical Rubber Co., 1966.

Davidsohn, Israel, and Wells, Benjamin B.: *Clinical Diagnosis by Laboratory Methods.* Philadelphia, W.B. Saunders, 1962.

Dubos, Rene J.: *Bacterial and Mycotic Infections of Man,* 3rd ed. Philadelphia, J.B. Lippincott, 1958.

Duemling, W.W.: Progressive disseminated coccidioidomycosis. *Arch Derm Syph, 60:*781-789, 1949.

Eckhoff, N.L.: Actinomycosis of the central nervous system: Report of two cases. *Lancet, 1:*7-8, 1941.

Emmons, C.W., Olson, B.J., and Eldridge, W.W.: Studies of the role of fungi in pulmonary disease. I. Cross reactions of histoplasmin. *Public Health Rep, 60:*1383-1394, 1945.

Fetter, Bernard F., Klintworth, Gorodn K., and Hendry, Wilson, S.: *Mycoses of the Central Nervous System.* Baltimore, Williams and Wilkins, 1967.

Fine, J.M., Franklin, D.A., and Lieberthol, A.S.: Mycotic meningitis due to *Candida albicans:* A four year recovery. *Neurology, 5:*438-443, 1953.

Fingegold, S.M., Will, D., and Murray, J.D.: Aspergillosis: A review and report of twelve cases. *Am J Med, 27:*463-482, 1959.

Frankel, Sam, Reitman, Stanley, and Sonnenwirth, Alex C.: *Gradwohl's Clinical Laboratory Methods and Diagnosis.* St. Louis, C.V. Mosby, 1963, Vol. I.

Frobisher, M., Jr.: *Fundamentals of Microbiology.* Philadelphia, W.B. Saunders, 1962.

Halpert, B., Whitcomb, F.C., McRoberts, C.C., and Carton, C.A.: Systemic and central nervous system involvement in crytococcosis and coccidioidomycosis. *Southern Med J, 47:*633-642, 1954.

Harvey, J.D., Cantrell, J.R., and Fisher, A.M.: Actinomycosis: Its recognition and treatment. *Ann Intern Med, 46:*868-885, 1957.

Heplar, Opal E.: *Manual of Clinical Laboratory Methods.* Springfield, Thomas, 1962.

Holmes, S.J., and Hawks, G.H.: Torulosis of the central nervous system. *Can Med Assoc J, 68*:143-146, 1953.

Jacobs, Morris B., Gerstein, Maurice J., and Walter, William G.: *Dictionary of Microbiology*. Princeton, N.J., D. Van Nostrand, 1957.

Jayewardene, R.P., and Wijekoon, W.B.: Cryptococcosis of the nervous system. *Postgrad Med J, 39*:546-547, 1963.

Jordon, Edwin O., and Burrows, William: *Textbook of Bacteriology*, 13th ed. Philadelphia and London, W.B. Saunders, 1941.

Keeney, Edmund L.: *Practical Medical Mycology*. Springfield, Thomas, 1955.

Khoo, T.K., Sugai, K., and Leong, T.K.: Disseminated aspergillosis: Case report and review of the world literature. *Amer J Clin Pathol, 45*:697-703, 1966.

Kolmer, John A., Spaulding, Earle H., and Robinson, Howard W.: *Approved Laboratory Technic*. New York, Appleton-Century-Crofts, 1951.

Kolmer, John A.: *Clinical Diagnosis by Laboratory Examinations*. New York, Appleton-Century-Crofts, 1944.

Krueger, E.G., Norso, L., Kenney, M., and Price, P.A.: Nocardiosis of the central nervous system. *J Neurosurg, 11*:226-233, 1954.

Laboratory Procedures in Clinical Mycology. Department of the Army, February, 1964.

Lacaz, C.S.: South American blastomycosis: A review. *Mycopathologia, 6*: 241-259, 1953.

Levinson, Samuel A., and MacFate, Robert P.: *Clinical Laboratory Diagnosis*. Philadelphia, Lee and Febiger, 1961.

Lewis, George M., and Hopper, Mary E.: *An Introduction to Medical Mycology*. Chicago, Year Book Publishers, 1948.

Lynch, Matthew J., Raphael, Stanley S., Mellor, Leslie D., Spare, Peter D., Hills, Peter, and Inwood, Martin: *Medical Laboratory Technology*. Philadelphia and London, W.B. Saunders, 1963.

McDowell, D.E., Ulmer, J.L., Velvo, A.G., Ekrem, W.S., and Kriz, J.P.: Cerebral abscesses due to *Actinomyces israeli*. *Southern Med J, 58*:227-230, 1965.

MacFate, Robert P.: *Introduction to the Clinical Laboratory*. Chicago, Year Book Medical Publishers, 1961.

Miller, Seward E.: *A Textbook of Clinical Pathology*. Baltimore, Williams and Wilkins, 1960.

Morgan, Rose M.: *Guide Questions for Medical Technology Examinations*. Springfield, Thomas, 1966.

Moss, Emma Sadler, and McQuown, Albert Louis: *Atlas of Medical Mycology*. Baltimore, Williams and Wilkins, 1953.

Nelson, J.S., Bates, R., and Pitchford, A.: Histoplasma meningitis. *Am J Dis Child, 102*:218-223, 1961.

Neter, Erwin, and Edgeworth, Dorothea Rae: *Medical Microbiology,* 4th ed. Philadelphia, F.A. Davis, 1962.

Parillo, O.J.: Disseminated mycotic disease. *JAMA, 114:*747-749, 1950.

Prior, J.A., Saslaw, S., and Cole, C.C.: Experiences with histoplasmosis. *Ann Intern Med, 40:*225-243, 1954.

Rankin, J., and Javid, M.: Nocardiosis of the central nervous system. *Neurology, 5:*815-820, 1955.

Rippey, J.J., Rober, W.A., Jeanes, A.L., and Bright, M.V.: Cryptococcal menigo-encephalitis. *J Clin Pathol, 18:*296-300, 1965.

Schulz, D.M.: Histoplasmosis of the central nerovus system. *JAMA, 151:* 549-551, 1953.

Schwartz, J.: Epidemologic study of North American blastomycosis. *Arch Dermatol, 71:*84-88, 1955.

Schwartz, J., and Baum, G.L.: Blastomycosis. *Am J Clin Pathol, 21:*999-1029, 1951.

Scott, Elvyn, Bailey, W. Robert, Schaub, Isabelle G., and Foley, M. Kathleen: *Diagnostic Bacteriology,* 5th ed. St. Louis, C.V. Mosby, 1958.

Sheppe, W.M.: Torula infection in man, 5th ed. *Am J Med Sci, 167:*91-108, 1924.

Smith, Alice Lorraine: *Principles of Microbiology,* 5th ed. St. Louis, C.V. Mosby, 1965.

Smith, Alice Lorraine: *Microbiology and Pathology,* 8th ed. St. Louis, C.V. Mosby, 1964.

Smith, C.E., Saito, M.T., and Simons, S.A.: Pattern of 39,500 serologic tests in coccidioidomycosis. *JAMA, 160:*546-552, 1956.

Smith, David T.: Zinnsser Microbiology, 13th ed. Appleton-Century-Crofts, 1964.

Todd, James Campbell, and Sanford, Arthur Hawley: *Clinical Diagnosis by Laboratory Methods.* Philadelphia and London, W.B. Saunders, 1943.

Tweten, L.: Cerebral mycosis: A clinico-pathological report of four cases. *Acta Neurol Scand, 41:*19-33, 1965.

Urdaneta, E., Pinto, V.B., and Gaveller, B.: Candidiasis. *Mycopathologica, 15:*317-342, 1961.

Waksman, Selman A.: *The Actinomyces.* New York, Ronald Press, 1967.

Weed, L.A., Anderson, H.A., Good, C.A., and Baggenstoss, A.H.: Nocardiosis: Clinical bacteriologic and pathologic aspects. *N Eng J Med, 253:*1137-1147, 1955.

Wells, Benjamin B.: *Clinical Pathology.* Philadelphia and London, W.B. Saunders, 1962.

Wells, Benjamin B.: *Clinical Pathology, Application, and Interpretation,* 2nd ed. Philadelphia and London, W.B. Saunders, 1956.

Wilson, G.S., and Miles, A.A.: *Topley and Wilson's Principles of Bacteri-*

ology and Immunity. Baltimore, Williams and Wilkins, 1955, Vols. I and II.

Wilson, J.W.: Cryptococcosis (Torulosis, European blastomycosis, Busse-Buschke's disease). *J Chronic Dis, 5:*445-459, 1957.

Zimmerman, L.E.: Total fungus infections complicating other diseases. *Am J Clin Pathol, 25:*46-65, 1955.

SECTION III

VIROLOGY

ARTHROPOD-BORNE (ARBOR) VIRUS
IDENTIFICATION

It is the responsibility of the nurse to assist the physician in obtaining the specimens and to transport these to the laboratory immediately after collection. *Strict aseptic precautions must be taken in all cases.*

PRINCIPLE OF THE TEST:

This group of viruses multiply in the bodies of arthropods. Viruses of this large group include *Group A,* containing Eastern and Western equine encephalomyelitis; *Group B* containing St. Louis encephalitis, Japanese B encephalitis, Murray Valley encephalitis, dengue fever, yellow fever, and louping ill. Group C contains Aspen, Marituba, and Oriboca. A miscellaneous group includes Rift Valley fever, Colorado tick fever, sandfly fever, and California encephalitis. A few examples are listed below.

Yellow Fever Virus: Isolation of the actual virus may be made from the blood or liver. Serologic tests such as the complement-fixation, virus neutralization, or hemagglutination-inhibition are of extreme importance. Animal inoculation, employing baby mice or monkeys, is frequently used.

Rift Valley Fever Virus: Acute-phase sera and convalescent-phase sera are tested for virus neutralizing antibodies and complement-fixing antibodies. Animal inoculation into the mouse, monkey, white rat, ferret, and hamster is of value. Tissue cultures derived from various animal species are employed with moderate success.

Dengue Virus: Antibody may be demonstrated by virus neutralization, hemagglutination-inhibition, and complement-fixation. Animal inoculation may include monkeys and mice.

Sandfly Fever Virus: Paired serum samples may be used for complement-fixation and virus neutralization tests. Animal inoculation, employing suckling mice, may be injected.

Colorado Tick Fever Virus: Animal inoculation, particularly of mice and hamsters, may be used. Chick embryo inoculation, employing the yolk sac, may also be used. The complement-fixation and virus neutralization tests are of value.

SPECIMEN REQUIRED:

Whole blood or paired sera samples (acute and convalescent) may be used; tissues such as the liver may be used.

PRESERVATIVE: None is permitted.

LENGTH OF TIME REQUIRED TO PERFORM TEST:
Animal Inoculation: Allow up to three weeks.
Serologic Tests: 24 to 48 hours.
Tissue Cultivation: Allow up to six weeks.
Egg Cultivation: three to four days.

NORMAL VALUES:

No pathogenic viruses isolated or identified by laboratory methods.

POSITIVE IN: Refer to *Principle of the Test.*

COXSACKIE VIRUS IDENTIFICATION

Nurses' Responsibility:

Strict aseptic technique must be employed in the collection and handling of all specimens, since droplet infection may take place through intermediary articles, fecal material, and other means. It may be the responsibility of the nurse to transport these specimens to the laboratory immediately after collection. Swabs and feces should be refrigerated at 4° to 6°C until sent to the laboratory. Cerebrospinal fluid must be kept frozen until it reaches the laboratory.

Principle of the Test:

Two distinct groups of Coxsackie viruses are known—Group A and Group B. Each group contains several immunologically distinct viruses.

Laboratory diagnosis of Coxsackie viruses is made by examining throat washing, stools, or cerebrospinal fluid. Virus neutralization tests are performed using paired sera and homologous virus. Cerebrospinal fluid or throat washings are used in their original state (with addition of antibiotics), while extracts of the stools are made by centrifuging the specimen at approximately 40,000 rpm. The sediment is then rendered free of bacteria by treatment with either antibiotics or ether.

Most Group A viruses are injected into seven-day old (or less) suckling mice, using peritoneal, cerebral, nasal, oral, intramuscular, or subcutaneous routes of injection. The mice are observed until they appear sick or paralyzed; they are then sacrificed, and histopathologic sections are made of the viscera, muscles, brain, and dorsal fat. Typing tests may be performed after the isolate has been passed through additional suckling mice. Group A causes myositis in suckling mice.

If Group B virus infections are suspected, 24-hour (or less) suckling mice are injected, or tissue cultivation procedures are utilized for typing of B strains. Virus neutralization, fluorescent antibody, histopathologic examination, and complement-fixation studies may be of value in establishing presumptive diagnosis. Fertile egg cultivation has not been widely used for Coxsackie viruses, since they do not grow readily. Tissue cultivation techniques are frequently employed and to a large extent have replaced animal inoculation methods. HeLa cell cultures and monkey kidney cell cultures are extensively used. Other laboratory animals which are often used for the isolation of Coxsackie viruses are suckling hamsters, chimpanzees, and cynomolgus monkeys.

SPECIMEN REQUIRED:

Clinical specimens include throat washings, swabs from mouth lesions or throat, stools, or cerebrospinal fluid. Paired serum samples, obtained before the fifth day and after the tenth day, may also be used.

PRESERVATIVE: None is permitted.

LENGTH OF TIME REQUIRED TO PERFORM TEST:

Allow up to four weeks for presumptive diagnosis.

NORMAL VALUES:

No pathogenic viruses of the Coxsackie group isolated. Coxsackie Group A viruses may be isolated from normal feces.

POSITIVE IN:

Aseptic meningitis, epidemic myalgia, epidemic pleurodynia, infantile myocarditis, herpangina, poliomyelitis.

EXANTHEMATA VIRUS IDENTIFICATION

It is the responsibility of the nurse to assist the physician in the collection of the specimens and to transport these to the laboratory immediately after collection.

PRINCIPLE OF THE TEST:

This group of viruses includes those causing measles (morbilli), German measles (rubella), roseola infantum, Boston exanthem, chickenpox (varicella), and smallpox (variola). The laboratory techniques for diagnosis of each of those viruses may differ.

Measles (Morbilli): Laboratory tests are rarely needed in the diagnosis of measles (Morbilli). However, at times, they may be of assistance. Virus neutralization tests may be performed on convalescent serum and in pooled samples of adult serum before infection. Other useful tests for the diagnosis of measles (morbilli) include tissue cultivation, egg inoculation, fluorescent antibody, and complement-fixation. Nasal smears of exudates may be stained and examined for giant Warthin-Finkeldey cells.

German Measles (Rubella): Laboratory tests are frequently of aid in the diagnosis of German measles (rubella). Blood or nasal washings may be inoculated into the monkey in laboratory experimentation. Tissue cultivation or chick embryo inoculation are frequently not successful.

Roseola Infantum (Exanthem Subitum): No etiologic agent has been isolated. The usual laboratory tests used for viral studies are not applicable to this disease.

Boston Exanthem: Virus neutralization are often performed on acute and convalescent sera.

Chickenpox (Varicella): It is rarely necessary for laboratory tests to be made to diagnose a case of chickenpox. Skin scrapings, made from the base of the vesicles, may be stained and examined for the characteristic giant cells. Tissue cultivation may also be of some value, as well as complement-fixation and tissue cultivation.

Smallpox: Laboratory diagnosis of smallpox may include egg cultivation, virus neutralization, complement-fixation, fluorescent

163

antibody, scrapings, animal inoculation, electron microscopy, histopathologic studies, flocculation (precipitation), agglutination, hemagglutination, and hemagglutination-inhibition. Demonstration of typical inclusions in the cytoplasm of Giemsa-stained cells may also assist in the diagnosis.

SPECIMEN REQUIRED:

Clinical specimens include serum, vesicle fluid, dried scabs, blood crusts, or scrapings from the lesion; serum before fifth day and after tenth day.

PRESERVATIVE: None is permitted.

LENGTH OF TIME REQUIRED TO PERFORM TEST:
Skin Scrapings: One hour.
Fluorescent Antibody: one to four hours.
Histopathologic Studies: 24 to 48 hours.
Serologic Studies: 24 hours.
Egg Cultivation: Three to four days.
Animal Inoculation: Allow up to three weeks.
Tissue Cultivation: Allow up to six weeks.

NORMAL VALUES:

No pathogenic viruses of the exanthemata group identified by laboratory methods.

POSITIVE IN: Refer to *Principle of the Test.*

GENITOURINARY VIRUS IDENTIFICATION

NURSES' RESPONSIBILITY:

It is the responsibility of the nurse to assist the physician in obtaining the specimens and to transport these to the laboratory immediately after collection.

PRINCIPLE OF THE TEST:

This group contains viruses responsible for causing herpes, inclusion cervicitis and urethritis, warts, and lymphogranuloma venereum.

Lymphogranuloma Venereum: Several laboratory tests are available for the diagnosis of lymphogranuloma venereum. Guinea pigs may be inoculated with bubo pus suspensions; mice (intracerebrally) and yolk sacs of embryonated eggs may be injected with the suspected material and examined for the characteristic Miyagawa's corpuscles. Direct smears are often made and stained by Giemsa's method. Histopathological studies are of value. The Frei test may be employed, as well as the complement-fixation test. Fluorescent antibody studies are of extreme value.

SPECIMEN REQUIRED:

Herpes: Vesicle fluid, crusts or scrapings from base of lesion, serum before fifth day and after tenth day.

Inclusion Cervicitis and Urethritis: Scrapings from cervix or urethra.

Warts: Entire tissue.

Lymphogranuloma venereum: Smears of pus for microscopic examination, pus from bubo for virus isolation, serum before tenth day and after fourteenth to twenty-first day, portions of lesion for histopathologic studies.

PRESERVATIVE: Formol-Zenker's solution (biopsy material) .

LENGTH OF TIME REQUIRED TO PERFORM TEST:
Microscopic Examination: One hour.
Virus Isolation: One to two months.
Serologic Tests: 24 hours.
Histopathologic Studies: 24 to 48 hours.

NORMAL VALUES:

No pathogenic viruses of this group isolated or identified by laboratory methods.

POSITIVE IN: Refer to *Principle of the Test.*

HEPATIC VIRUS IDENTIFICATION

NURSES' RESPONSIBILITY:

It is the responsibility of the nurse to assist the physician in obtaining the specimens and to transport these to the laboratory immediately after collection. *Strict aseptic precautions must be taken at all times when obtaining the specimens.*

PRINCIPLE OF THE TEST:

This group contains viruses which cause infectious hepatitis (virus A) and homologous serum jaundice (virus B).

Infectious Hepatitis: Animal inoculation is *not* applicable to isolation of this virus since it is not pathogenic for any known laboratory animal. Blood sera have revealed isolation of the virus during the *acute* phase of the disease. Duodenal contents may be used, in which the virus is demonstrated three days before onset and in the acute phase.

Homologous Serum Jaundice: Animal inoculation is *not* applicable to isolation of this virus since it is not pathogenic for any known laboratory animal. Egg cultivation is not used. Human volunteers are used for experimental purposes.

SPECIMEN REQUIRED:

The viruses have been shown to be present in serum, whole blood, red blood cells, plasma, fibrinogen, and thrombin.

PRESERVATIVE: None is permitted.

LENGTH OF TIME REQUIRED TO PERFORM TEST:

Serologic Testing: 24 to 48 hours.

NORMAL VALUES:

The icterogenic viruses occur in the serum of a number of healthy and apparently normal individuals.

POSITIVE IN: Infectious hepatitis and homologous serum jaundice.

167

NEUROTROPIC VIRUS IDENTIFICATION

NURSES' RESPONSIBILITY:

It is the responsibility of the nurse to assist the physician in obtaining the specimens and to transport these to the laboratory immediately after collection. *Strict aseptic precautions must be taken at all times when working with these materials.* Clinical specimens include nervous tissue, cerebrospinal fluid, stools, throat secretions, and paired sera samples. If *nervous tissue* is used, the brain and spinal cord are removed by aseptic technique and parts of the spinal cord, cerebral cortex, basal ganglia, hippocampus, and brain stem are divided into three parts each, which are treated as follows. One part is placed in 50% sterile glycerol in saline and stored at 4° to 6° C; one part stored in a carbon dioxide refrigerator at −60°C; and one part placed in formalin for histopathologic sections.

If *cerebrospinal fluid* is used, one part is sent to the laboratory for chemical, bacteriological, and cytological tests, and one part is frozen at −60° C for further testing if necessary.

Stools and *throat secretions* are collected and frozen at −60°C until used. Two or three consecutive stools should be collected in screw cap containers, and washings of throat swabbings or nasopharyngeal secretions are stored at −60°C.

Acute and *convalescent sera* samples are needed to obtain comparative antibody levels. Convalescent-phase sera is most often obtained 10 to 14 days after the onset of the disease. A three-month blood sample may be taken for follow-up studies. All sera samples are removed from the clot as soon after collection as possible, and kept frozen at −60°C with no heat inactivation.

PRINCIPLE OF THE TEST:

This group contains viruses responsible for causing virus meningitis (aseptic meningitis), poliomyelitis and poliomyelitis-like illnesses, rabies, and encephalitis. Inocula may be prepared and injected into animals or eggs, and used for tissue cultivation.

Preparation of inocula for the various laboratory tests may

168

differ. *Brain* and *cord tissue* is ground in a mortar, and a 1:10 suspension in sterile saline (containing antibiotics) is made. The suspension is centrifuged and the supernatant fluid used for animal and egg inoculation tests. Tissue cultures of brain and cord tissue may be made, employing monkey kidney, human amnion, or HeLa cells. *Stools* may be suspended in water and centrifuged at 3000 rpm. for about 20 minutes, the deposit treated with ether, and a small suspension in saline (containing antibiotics) made for inoculation.

Throat washings are usually treated with antibiotics prior to inoculation, while *cerebrospinal fluid* may be inoculated without any prior treatment. *Serologic tests* for neurotropic virus infections most often include virus neutralization, complement-fixation, and fluorescent antibody tests.

Virus Meningitis (Aseptic Meningitis): This group contains viruses causing infections such as Coxsackie Group B meningitis, leptospirosis, mump meningitis, ECHO meningitis, and lymphocytic choriomeningitis. Animal inoculation and serologic tests, such as agglutination, complement-fixation, virus neutralization, and fluorescent antibody, may be used in the diagnosis of virus meningitis (aseptic meningitis) .

Poliomyelitis Illnesses: Animal inoculation is one of the more frequently used methods for identification of the poliomyelitis virus. Rhesus monkeys *(Macaca mulatta)* are injected with the poliomyelitis virus, employing the cerebral route. Direct intraneural, intraspinal, nasal instillation, inhalation of atomized particles of virus, and intraperitoneal, intramuscular, or intradermal routes of injection are frequently employed. Chimpanzees are often used as laboratory animals. Tissue cultivations, employing many techniques, are extremely valuable in the study of the poliomyelitis virus. The virus is most often recovered from feces or throat washings. Virus neutralization tests on paired sera are frequently performed on tissue cultures. Fluorescent antibody studies are of extreme value.

Poliomyelitis-like Illnesses: Viruses such as Coxsackie, ECHO, and "Iceland disease," may simulate the poliomyelitis virus. Diagnoses is accomplished in the same manner as described for the poliomyelitis virus.

Rabies: The rabies virus may be identified by injecting saliva or brain tissue containing the virus intracerebrally into mice. Seller's stained slides and fluorescent antibody studies are also employed. Refer to *Rabies Virus Identification,* page 174, for a complete description.

Virus Encephalitis: Several varieties of encephalitis, which include sporadic encephalitis, postinfectious and postvaccination encephalitis, encephalitis lethargica, North American equine encephalitis: Eastern and Western types, St. Louis encephalitis, Venezuelan equine encephalitis, Japanese B encephalitis, and tickborne encephalitis. Hemagglutination studies, animal inoculation, fluorescent antibody, histopathological studies, virus neutralization, agglutination, tissue cultivation, complement-fixation, and egg inoculation may be used in the diagnosis.

SPECIMEN REQUIRED:

 Virus Meningitis: Cerebrospinal fluid, serum or citrated blood collected at the onset of illness and also 21 to 40 days later.

 Poliomyelitis: Histopathological sections of the central nervous system, such as the pons, medulla, motor cortex, and basal ganglia, stools, throat washings or swabs, cerebrospinal fluid, serum before third day and after tenth day.

 Rabies: Portions of hippocampus, saliva.

 Virus Encephalitis: Serum before fourteenth day, brain tissue, cerebrospinal fluid.

PRESERVATIVE:

 Central Nervous System Tissue: 50% sterile glycerol in saline; formalin.

NORMAL VALUES:

No pathogenic viruses of this group isolated or identified by laboratory methods.

LENGTH OF TIME REQUIRED TO PERFORM TEST:

 Virus Meningitis: Virus isolation— four to twenty days.

 *Poliomyelitis and Poliomyelitis-like illnesses—*Virus isolation— ten days, serologic tests—one to fifteen days.

Rabies: Virus isolation—seven to fourteen days, Negri body examination—one to five days.

Virus Encephalitis: Virus isolation—one to ten days, serologic tests—up to thirty days.

POSITIVE IN: Refer to Principle of the Test.

OPHTHALMIC VIRUS IDENTIFICATION

NURSES' RESPONSIBILITY:

Extreme care must be exercised in the handling of all clinical specimens. It is the responsibility of the nurse to assist the physician in the collection of specimens and to transport these to the laboratory immediately after the collection.

PRINCIPLE OF THE TEST:

This group of viruses includes those that cause trachoma, epidemic keratoconjunctivitis, herpetic keratitis, inclusion conjunctivitis, and Newcastle virus conjunctivitis. Numerous laboratory tests are available in the isolation and identification of this group of viruses.

Trachoma: Superficial conjunctival scrapings are placed on a glass slide; the slide is fixed in alcohol, stained with a 1:20 solution of Giemsa's stain for 24 hours, examined microscopically for the characteristic Halberstaedter-Prowazek inclusions in epithelial cells. Egg inoculation is at times desirable although not as successful. Complement-fixation and skin tests have been shown to be unreliable.

Epidemic Keratoconjunctivitis: Eye scrapings may be cultured in HeLa cells. Virus neutralization tests are also used.

Inclusion Conjunctivitis: Scrapings of the cervix, urethra, or conjunctiva are spread thinly on slides; the slides are "fixed" in alcohol, stained with dilute Giemsa's stain or by Gram's method and are examined for the characteristic basophilic granular inclusions (Thygeson bodies). Egg inoculation, although occasionally used, is still considered unsuccessful.

Newcastle Virus Conjunctivitis: An aliquot of the conjunctival exudate, blood, or throat washings (treated with antibiotics) is often inoculated into embryonated eggs. Virus neutralization, hemagglutination-inhibition, and complement-fixation tests are often employed.

SPECIMEN REQUIRED:

Trachoma: Smears or scrapings from tarsal conjunctiva, lesions, or serum before tenth day and after fourteenth day; eye washings may be used.

172

Epidemic Keratoconjunctivitis: Scrapings from eye, throat and eye washings, paired sera.

Inclusion Conjunctivitis: Scrapings from conjunctiva, eye and throat washings, paired sera.

Newcastle Virus Conjunctivitis: Eye or throat washings, conjunctival exudates, paired sera.

LENGTH OF TIME REQUIRED TO PERFORM TESTS:

Microscopic Examination: One hour.

Egg Inoculation: Three to four days.

Serologic Tests: 24-48 hours .

NORMAL VALUES:

No pathogenic viruses isolated or identified by laboratory methods.

POSITIVE IN: Refer to *Principle of the Test.*

RABIES VIRUS IDENTIFICATION

SYNONYMS: Seller's Test, Negri Body Test.

NURSES' RESPONSIBILITY:

No special preparation of the patient is needed. Rubber gloves *must* be worn at all times in handling of the specimens.

PRINCIPLE OF THE TEST:

The rabies virus is considered to be one of the most highly neurotropic viruses. An inclusion body, known as the *negri body,* is pathognomonic of rabies. It is found in the ganglion cells of Ammon's horn (hippocampus major), the pyramidal cell layer of the cerebral cortex, in cerebral nerve nuclei, in basal ganglia, and in the Purkinje cell layer of the cerebellum.

The animal suspected of harboring the rabies virus is permitted to die a natural death, since negri bodies develop as the disease progresses. If the animal is sacrificed too early, the negri bodies may not be demonstrable. If the animal is living after 14 days, it may be assumed that it is not infected with the rabies virus. It is important to realize that the animal is considered infected with the rabies virus until negative tests are proven valid.

The head of the animal suspected of harboring the rabies virus is removed and tissue impressions or smears made from the above mentioned tissues. An aniline dye, such as methylene blue or Seller's stain, is used to stain the tissue. Seller's stain shows the negri bodies as *bright red* structures with blue internal granules; methylene blue stain shows the negri bodies as a *light red* with basophilic granules.

Isolation of the virus may be accomplished by intracerebral inoculation of mice. Six or eight mice are injected intracerebrally with approximately 0.03 ml of 10% brain emulsion from the suspected animal. Saliva may also be used. The inoculated mice are observed for a maximum of 30 days from the initial injection. If the brain suspension contains the rabies virus, the animals will die within seven to ten days. Death that occurs within the first 48 hours is considered to be due to some other cause. The mice showing symptoms of rabies are then sacrificed; the brains are removed and examined for rabies by the previously mentioned methods.

SPECIMEN REQUIRED:

A tissue impression and/or smear from the hippocampus of the suspected material is needed; saliva may be used.

PRESERVATIVE:

If the tissue is to be sent to another laboratory, it should be preserved with either glycerin or saline, or by freezing with dry ice and packing in a stout metal container. When fluorescent antibody tests are to be performed, the tissue impressions are "fixed" in acetone for a minimum of 30 minutes and kept refrigerated until tested.

LENGTH OF TIME REQUIRED TO PERFORM TEST:

Depending on the method used, it may take as long as 30 days for the report.

NORMAL VALUES:

Tissue Impressions: On smears stained with Seller's, methylene blue, Giemsa, etc; no negri bodies found.

Fluorescent Antibody Test: Negative.

Neutralization Test: Negative.

Mouse Inoculation: No death of animals 10 to 30 days after inoculation.

POSITIVE IN: Rabies.

RESPIRATORY VIRUS IDENTIFICATION

NURSES' RESPONSIBILITY:

It is the responsibility of the nurse to assist the physician in obtaining the specimens and to transport these to the laboratory immediately after the collection. *All materials must be handled with aseptic precautions.*

PRINCIPLE OF THE TEST:

This group of viruses contains mumps, adenoviruses, the common cold, influenza, virus pneumonia, basophilic virus-causing pneumonitis, psittacosis and ornithosis, primary atypical pneumonia, infantile virus pneumonia, cytomegalic inclusion disease, and acute laryngotracheobronchitis.

Numerous laboratory identification methods are available for the diagnosis of this group of viruses.

Mumps: Saliva, which has been collected by either mechanical aspirator or swabs placed near the orifices of Stensen's ducts, is injected (with antibiotics) into eight-day chick embryos; five days later the amniotic fluid is withdrawn and hemagglutination tests are done. Virus neutralization tests with known antisera, tissue cultivation, complement-fixation, hemagglutination-inhibition, and red cell agglutination tests are also utilized in diagnosis. Cerebrospinal fluid, urine, or acute and convalescent-phase sera may be used. Fluorescent antibody tests are of extreme value.

Adenoviruses: Diagnosis is often made by inoculation of HeLa cell or human amnion tissue cultures. Complement-fixation tests with a known antiserum may also be run on any isolated adenovirus on both acute and convalescent sera. Virus neutralization tests are of some value, and fluorescent antibody tests are of extreme value.

Common Cold: Diagnosis of the common cold rarely requires laboratory testing. If viral isolation is desired, bacteria-free filtrates of nasal washings are injected into chimpanzees. Tissue cultivation may be used as well as complement-fixation tests.

Influenza: Tissue cultivation, employing minced chick embryo or embryonic membranes suspended in nutritive fluids, is most frequently used for the isolation of influenza viruses. Hemagglutination tests are performed on the isolate. Egg cultivation and animal inoculation may be of value. Numerous serologic tests may be of value, among which are flocculation, virus neutralization, fluorescent antibody, complement-fixation, and hemagglutination-inhibition.

"Virus pneumonia": This includes several viruses all of which cause pulmonary lesions. These are measles, mumps, psittacosis, ornithosis, Eaton agent pneumonia (primary atypical pneumonia), and lymphocytic choriomeningitis. Animal inoculation, particularly of mice by nasal or peritoneal routes of injection, and frequently hamsters or cotton rats, may be used. Ferrets are often inoculated nasally. Fertile egg inoculations are also employed, using the yolk sac for the route of injection. Hemagglutination studies may be performed on the isolates. Complement-fixation tests are also of some value, as are histopathologic studies.

Basophilic Virus Pneumonitis: This group contains viruses causing pneumonitis in man, such as psittacosis, ornithosis, and lymphogranuloma venereum. Other viruses included in this group include meningopneumonitis virus, pneumonia virus of mice, San Francisco virus, and The Louisiana and Illinois virus. Animal inoculation of mice, hamsters, guinea pigs, cotton rats, and pigeons is of great value in identifying members of this group. Other valuable tests include toxin neutralization, virus neutralization, and cross-immunity tests in mice. Complement-fixation tests with absorbed sera are sometimes used to advantage.

Psittacosis and Ornithosis: Clinical specimens, such as blood, lung tissue, or sputum, are inoculated intranasally or intraperitoneally into the yolk sac of embryonated eggs. Complement-fixation tests, employing serum taken at the onset of the disease and also at ten to fourteen days after onset, may be used. Histopathological and direct microscopical studies may also reveal significant changes.

Primary Atypical Pneumonia: Paired samples of blood serum (acute and convalescent), are tested for cold agglutinins and *streptococcus* MG agglutinins, as well as for the actual organism (Eaton agent). Other tests for the diagnosis of primary "atypical" pneumonia include fluorescent antibody, fertile egg cultivation, tissue cultivation, culture, agglutination, hemagglutination, hemagglutination-inhibition, hemolytic plaque, and tetrazolium reduction tests. Refer to *Eaton Agent Identification,* page 40, for a complete description.

Infantile Virus Pneumonia: Nasal inoculation of mice with suspected virus-containing material is often employed. Hemagglutination studies of the isolate may aid in the diagnosis.

Cytomegalic Inclusion Disease: Histopathological studies may be run on almost all of the viscera, such as lungs, thyroid, liver, brain, bone marrow, testes, and kidney.

Acute Laryngotracheobronchitis: Tissue cultivation on monkey kidney cells, human amniotic cells, and HeLa cells may be used. Hemagglutination studies are also of value.

SPECIMEN REQUIRED:

Mumps: Saliva; cerebrospinal fluid, urine, or serum before the sixth day and after the fourteenth day; brain, spinal cord (at autopsy).

Adenovirus: Throat swabs, swabs from conjunctiva, serum before fifth and after tenth day, lung tissue (at autopsy).

Common Cold: Nasal washings (bacterial-free filtrates).

Influenza: Throat swabs and washings, serum before third day and after tenth day; lung (biopsy).

"Virus Pneumonia": Saliva, cerebrospinal fluid, serum before sixth and after fourteenth day.

Basophilic Virus Pneumonitis: Sputum, cerebrospinal fluid, serum before third day and after tenth day.

Psittacosis and Ornithosis: Sputum, citrated blood, serum before third and after tenth day.

Primary Atypical Pneumonia: Sputum, pharyngeal swab, serum before tenth day and after fourteenth day, throat washings.

Infantile Virus Pneumonia: Saliva, cerebrospinal fluid, serum before sixth and after fourteenth day.

Cytomegalic Inclusion Disease: Viscera, saliva, urine, paired sera.

Acute Laryngotracheobronchitis: Throat washings.

PRESERVATIVE: None required.

LENGTH OF TIME REQUIRED TO PERFORM TEST:

Fluorescent Antibody: One to four hours.

Histopathologic Studies: 24 to 48 hours.

Serologic Studies: 24 hours.

Egg Cultivation: Three to four days.

Tissue Cultivation: Up to four weeks.

NORMAL VALUES:

No pathogenic viruses of the respiratory group isolated or identified by laboratory methods.

POSITIVE IN: Refer to *Principle of the Test.*

SKIN OR MUCOUS MEMBRANES VIRUS
IDENTIFICATION

Nurses' Responsibility:

It is the responsibility of the nurse to assist the physician in the collection of the specimens and to transport these to the laboratory immediately after collection.

Principle of the Test:

This group contains viruses causing molluscum contagiosum, warts (verrucae), foot and mouth disease, contagious pustular dermatitis (Ecthyma), herpes zoster, and herpes simplex.

Molluscum Contagiosum: Numerous laboratory tests may be employed in the identification of this virus, including electron microscopy and histopathologic studies. Diagnosis is often added by mounting an exudate wet in liquor potassii or Lugol's iodine and examining for inclusions. Paschen's or Giemsa's method may be used to stain the films for elementary bodies.

Warts (Verrucae): Histopathological and electron microscopy are of value. Inoculation of the virus may be accomplished by tissue cultivation methods.

Foot-and-Mouth Disease: Isolation of the virus may be made in the foot pad of the guinea pig or intraperitoneally in suckling mice. Acute phase sera and convalescent-phase sera may be employed for virus neutralization and complement-fixation tests.

Contagious Pustular Dermatitis (Ecthyma): The virus may be grown in the skin of guinea pigs, sheep, and rabbits, but it is difficult to propagate in chick embryos. Electron microscopy is an important aid in the diagnosis. Cross-immunity tests are of value in the identification.

Herpes Zoster (Shingles): Diagnosis of herpes zoster is comparatively easy and most often requires no laboratory aids. Animal and egg inoculations may be employed using vesicle fluid. Cytology studies, such as smears from the lesions, may be of some value. Tissue cultivation, employing human embryonic tissue, may be employed.

Herpes Simplex (Febrilis): Scrapings of the base of the herpetic lesion often are placed on a slide or coverslip and stained by Giemsa's stain or hematoxylin and eosin. The preparations are then examined for the characteristic Tzanck giant cells. Isolation of the virus may be made from pathologic specimens by tissue cultivation methods employing human tissues, HeLa cells, or rabbit kidney or cornea. Inoculation of suckling mice may be used. Egg inoculation, employing chorioallantoic membranes, may also be used. Fluorescent antibody studies are of extreme value.

SPECIMEN REQUIRED:

Molluscum Contagiosum: Vesicle fluid from the node.

Warts (Verrucae): Entire tissue.

Foot-and-Mouth Disease: Vesicle fluid of lesion.

Contagious Pustular Dermatitis (Ecthyma): Vesicular fluid.

Herpes Zoster (Shingles): Vesicle fluid, serum before fifth day and after tenth day.

Herpes Simplex (Febrilis): Vesicle fluid, crusts or scrapings from base of lesion, serum before fifth day and after tenth day.

PRESERVATIVE:

Often no preservative is needed. However, in herpes simplex (febrilis) the brain may be preserved frozen or in glycerol-saline.

LENGTH OF TIME REQUIRED TO PERFORM TEST:

Histopathologic Studies: 24 to 48 hours.

Serologic Tests: 24 hours.

Microscopic Examination: Two to twelve hours.

Tissue Cultivation: Allow up to six weeks.

Egg Inoculation: Three to four days.

Fluorescent Antibody: One to four hours.

NORMAL VALUES:

No pathologic viruses of this group isolated or identified by laboratory methods.

POSITIVE IN: Refer to *Principle of the Test.*

VIRAL STUDIES

Viruses are organisms which parasitize man, animals, bacteria, insects, and plants; they require both living and intracellular enzymes for growth. Viruses behave as living agents, and they are of minute size with a relatively simple chemical structure. The system of viral classification has long been disputed, and it appears that it will be some years before a concrete classification will be established. The authors of this book have described the virus identification of man according to the *system* predominantly affected, i.e. the respiratory viruses, hepatic viruses, etc., and it is to be remembered that the laboratory tests must always be assessed in relation to the clinical picture. The reader is referred to the individual descriptions of viral diagnoses listed alphabetically as follows:

Arthroped-borne Virus Identification, p. 159.
Coxsackie Virus Identification, p. 161.
Exanthemata Virus Identification, p. 163.
Genitourinary Virus Identification, p. 165.
Hepatic Virus Identification, p. 167.
Neurotropic Virus Identification, p. 168.
Ophthalmic Virus Identification, p. 172.
Rabies Virus Identification, p. 174.
Respiratory Virus Identification, p. 176.
Skin or Mucous Membranes Virus Identification, p. 180.

Laboratory Diagnosis: Laboratory diagnosis of viral diseases includes many different techniques, such as agglutination, animal inoculation, electron microscopy, fertile egg cultivation, fluorescent antibody, skin tests, tissue cultivation, and serologic tests such as hemagglutination, hemagglutination-inhibition, precipitation (flocculation), and virus neutralization. A brief description of each of these laboratory tests is presented.

Animal Inoculation: Animal inoculation is the oldest method of virus cultivation. The animal chosen and the route of injection will depend largely on the suspected virus. Numerous laboratory animals are used for the isolation of viruses, among which are guinea pigs, mice, rats, rabbits, monkeys, chimpanzees, rabbits, and ferrets. Suckling mice are the most frequently used. Refer to *Animal Inoculation*, page 9 for a more detailed description.

Electron Microscopy: The electron microscope, with its potential of magnifying an object up to $\times$ 5,000,000 with good definition, has greatly facilitated the study of viruses, and although the electron microscope is not an instrument in routine use, it does have some practical application in cases where the virus may not be seen with the ordinary light microscope.

Fertile Egg Cultivation: Chick embryos of five to fifteen days are used for viral study and propagation because of the many advantages. This technique is less expensive, less time consuming, requires less volume of space, is less hazardous to workers, and shows evidence of a lesser degree of cross-infection. For these reasons, eggs are usually preferred to former methods of ainmal inoculation for propagation of viruses.

Dark-shelled eggs are usually *not* used because they are difficult to candle. White Leghorn eggs are most often preferred by virologists, although turkey and duck eggs, guinea fowl, and pigeon eggs are also utilized. The eggs are preincubated at 10° to 15°C, and then incubated at 38° to 39°C with a relative humidity between 55 to 60%. After the eggs have been incubated, they are examined to assure life of the embryo prior to inoculation. The egg is candled by placing it over a box containing a 100 watt lamp in a darkened room. The air sac, the position of the embryo, and the major blood vessels are then marked prior to the innoculation. The egg is drilled in the desired spot, using either a dental drill or a diamond steel disc.

After the inoculum is injected, the drilled groove is sealed by means of a wax mixture. The eggs are candled every day until death of the embryo, at which time the fluids are collected in the following manner: The eggs are chilled at refrigerator temperatures of 4° to 6°C for four to six hours. The wax seal over the site of the inoculation is opened, and the fluid is pipetted out with a Pasteur pipette drawn to a fine tip. The fluid is then cultured. Routes of inoculation most commonly employed are the following:

Allantoic Cavity: This route employs nine- to twelve-day eggs. The quantity of inoculum used is approximately 0.1 to 0.2 ml, which is injected by means of a tuberculin syringe and needle, or by a dissecting needle into the allantoic sac through a hole previously drilled in the side of the egg.

Amniotic Cavity: This route employs seven-to fifteen-day eggs. The quantity of inoculum is 0.1 to 0.2 ml, which is injected onto the amniotic membrane by means of a tuberculin syringe and needle. This technique is usually the choice in primary isolation of the influenza virus.

Chorioallantoic Membrane: This route employs ten- to twelve-day embryos. The quantity of inoculum used is 0.1 to 0.5 ml, which is injected onto the chorioallantoic membrane. The inoculation is most often made with a graduated Pasteur pipette drawn out to a fine tip. An artificial air sac is created by puncturing the air sac and shell to ensure efficiency of the inoculation. The eggs are incubated in a horizontal position. Virus infections characterized by focal lesions, such as those of the pox viruses, are most frequently inoculated into the chorioallantoic membrane.

Yolk Sac: This route employs five- to eight-day embryos. The quantity of inoculum is 0.2 to 1.0 ml, which is injected by tuberculin syringe and needle into the yolk sac. The yolk sac is susceptible to all known viruses and rickettsiae.

Intracerebral: This route employs eight- to fourteen-day embryos. The quantity of inoculum is 0.01 to 0.02 ml, which is injected via tuberculin syringe and needle.

Fluorescent Antibody: The fluorescent antibody test is of great aid in the demonstration of viral antigens, such as those of the rabies virus (refer to *Rabies Virus Identification,* p. 174), and is rapidly growing in stature as a diagnostic tool in the diagnosis of diseases of bacteriologic, parasitic, viral, and rickettsial nature.

Skin Tests: Skin tests are of value in the diagnosis of viral diseases such as cat-scratch disease and Lymphogranuloma venereum.

Tissue Cultivation: Tissue cultivation has shown itself to be one of the most successful means for the study of viruses in man and animals. Among the currently used animal tissues are monkey kidney tissues, human amnion tissues, and commercially available cell lines such as those of the HeLa cells.

Monkey Kidney Cell Culture: Kidney "monolayer" cultures are most frequently used for the isolation of poliomyelitis, "ECHO", and Coxsackie viruses from pathologic materials.

Either one or both kidneys of an adult monkey is removed aseptically, and is decapsulated and incised transversely. The pelvis and adhering connecting tissue are removed. The kidney tissue is minced, washed with physiologic saline, Hank's solution, or a growth medium containing antibodies.

Preheated (37°C) 0.25% trypsin, in a balanced salt solution, is added to the tissue in a trypsinization flask to liberate epithelial cells. The suspension is heated at 37°C for 30 minutes, and the process is repeated three times. The suspension is centrifuged and the cell pellets from the sediment placed in a growth medium and incubated at 37°C until inoculated. After inoculation, the tubes are placed horizontally in a stationary rack for seven to ten days until a profuse growth of epithelial cells occurs, usually one layer thick—hence the term, "monolayer." The areas of necrosis or "plaques" are counted, each "plaque" representing one elementary body.

Human Amnion Cell Culture: Human placental tissue is obtained aseptically from a maternity ward after a natural delivery or from a Caesarean section, if at all possible. *Great care must be taken to avoid trauma of the tissue.* As soon as the tissue is obtained, it is placed in Hank's solution and transported to the laboratory. The amnion must be processed within ten hours after the collection in the same way as that for monkey kidney cell culture described above.

HeLa Cell Culture: HeLa cells, originally derived from a carcinoma of the cervix, are available from commercial sources for the isolation of most viruses and are processed much in the same way as for those of monkey kidney cells.

Serologic Tests: Serologic testing is a widely used diagnostic aid in viral diseases. Several different tests are available for measuring antibody titers. Among the tests are agglutination, cold agglutinins, complement-fixation, hemadsorption, hemagglutination, hemagglutination-inhibition, precipitation (flocculation), and virus neutralization. All serologic tests are carefully correlated with the clinical picture for proper evaluation. A serial four-fold rise in titer between the acute phase serum and the convalescent phase serum is considered significant.

Agglutination: Certain viruses, when combined with serum containing specific antibodies, cause specific agglutination (clumping) to occur. These aggregates may be seen either macroscopically or microscopically. Among the viral diseases in which agglutination tests have been shown to be successful are vaccinia, varicella, herpes zoster, influenza, and psittacosis. The agglutination test is little employed in viral diagnostic work.

Cold Agglutinins: Cold agglutinins are found in elevated titers in certain viral conditions, such as primary "atypical" pneumonia. Serum of the patient is placed with Group "O" red cells, placed in a refrigerator at 0° to 5°C, and observed for agglutination, indicating "cold agglutinins" are present.

Complement-Fixation: The complement-fixation test employs complement, a chemical substance present in normal serum, that is absorbed by any combination of antigen with antibody. A hemolytic indicator system, which consists of sheep erythrocytes and a heated antiserum against the erythrocytes, is used to detect the final presence or absence of complement. Complement-fixation antibodies most often appear in the serum during the first to third weeks of onset of illness; they then rise to a plateau, and fall in five to six months, finally disappearing within twelve to eighteen months. Viruses contain two antigenic components that fix complement: soluble antigen, and virus antigen or elementary body.

Hemadsorption: This procedure is used for detecting viruses grown in tissue culture. Certain viruses produce hemagglutinin, which in turn adsorbs erythrocytes to cell surfaces in which the virus has grown. A washed sheep-cell suspension is added to a viral culture. Formation of rosettes (and clusters by the erythrocytes) around the infected cells of the viral culture is observed microscopically.

Hemagglutination: Most of the disease-producing viruses have the capacity, either by direct or indirect action, to agglutinate red blood cells. Agglutination may occur with the red cells of many animals, such as human Group "O" fowl, guinea pigs, and chickens. Union of erythrocytes which possess receptors with the virus produces a change in the erythrocytes, causing them to agglutinate.

Hemagglutination-Inhibition: Antibodies of some viruses have the ability to inhibit agglutination of erythrocytes. The hemagglutination-inhibition test is frequently used in the identification of specific strains of a virus, such as the influenza virus. Serial dilutions of the patient's serum are added to viral antigen; the tubes are incubated, washed erythrocytes are added, and the tubes are then observed for agglutination. Suspensions of certain viruses cause red blood cells of various animal species to agglutinate, but if specific immune serum is added, the agglutination will be inhibited proportionately to the amount of antibody in the patient's serum. A fourfold increase in titer between the acute-phase serum and convalescent-phase serum is considered significant.

Precipitation (flocculation): This technique is used primarily in connection with the variola-vaccinia group of viruses. Aqueous tissue extracts contain a heat-labile and heat-stable viral antigen which, when in contact with a specific antiserum, causes a precipitation (flocculation) reaction to occur.

Virus Neutralization: The virus neutralization test is based on the neutralization of infectious viruses by specific virus-neutralizing antibodies. Two chief uses of the tests are: (1) to detect specific elevated rises in antibody, and (2) to identify the viral isolate. Neutralization tests are primarily used in the diagnoses of neurotropic and Coxsackie virus infections.

Collection of Specimens: Various diseases caused by viruses require different sources of materials for isolation and serologic tests. Frequently used clinical materials include feces, vesicle exudates, throat washings, blood, and cerebrospinal fluid. Tissue biospy and autopsy tissues are often used. Collection, storage, and transport of specimens are essential in the successful identification of any virus. All virus isolation materials require *immediate* freezing at temperatures of −20° to −70°C.

Feces: Feces collected for viral studies must be collected in a satisfactory container, preferably a sterile, wide-mouthed bottle. Immediately after collection, the specimens are frozen at −60°C. Refer to *Feces Collection,* page 45. If specimens are to be shipped to another laboratory, dry ice is often used. Anal swabs may be used and are often placed in a tube of broth and frozen, or in a tube containing 50% glycerin-saline.

Blood and Cerebrospinal Fluid: Blood specimens used for viral studies are most often heparinized or citrated, although sera is frequently used. Spinal fluid may be used without prior treatment. Refer to *Blood Culture,* page 23, and *Cerebrospinal Fluid Collection,* page 31.

Tissue Specimens: Tissue specimens are obtained aseptically at biopsy or at autopsy and are placed in sterile containers. Tissue specimens are most often stored at −60°C. If tissues are to be inoculated into embryonated eggs or animals, they are finely ground in a mortar, using an abrasive. Antibiotics are at times added to prevent bacterial growth.

Throat Washings: Throat washings are collected as early in the course of disease as possible. Refer to *Throat Culture,* page 96.

Skin Lesions or Mucous Membranes: Cotton swabs are used to collect exudates from lesions, such as those in smallpox or vaccinia. The swabs are placed in a holding broth and are then frozen, or placed in 50% glycerin-saline.

VIRUSES — NOMENCLATURE

Certain viruses are known to clinicians by various terminology. The following is a listing of the preferred names of the various viruses, as well as some of the most commonly known synonyms.

VIRUSES—PREFERRED NAMES AND SYNONYMS

PREFERRED NAME	SYNONYM(S)
Adenoviruses	APC, ARD, and RI viruses.
Common Cold Virus	*Tarpeia premens* spec. nov.
Common Wart Virus	*Molitor verrucae,* verricae virus, virus papillomateux, Warzen-Virus.
ECHO Viruses	ECHO—cytopathogenic, enteric, human, orphan.
Encephalitis Lethargic Virus	A Encephalitis virus.
Equine Encephalitis Viruses (Western, Eastern, Venezuelan)	*Erro equinus,* equine encephalo-myelitis virus.
Foot and Mouth Disease Virus	*Hostis pecoris.*
Hepatitis Virus A	Virus of infectious hepatitis.
Hepatitis Virus B	Virus of serum hepatitis.
Herpes Virus	*Herpesvirus hominis, Neuro-cystitis herpetii, Scelus recurrens,* virus of herpes simplex (febrilis) .
Herpesvirus simiae	B Virus.
Influenza A Virus	*Tarpeia alpha* spec. nov.
Influenza B Virus	*Tarpeia beta* spec. nov.
Japanese B Encephalitis Virus	*Erro japonicus.*
Louping Ill Virus	*Erro scoticus,* virus of sheep encephalitis.
Lymphocytic Choriomeningitis Virus	*Legio erbea* spec. nov.
Measles Virus	*Briareus morbillorum,* Masern-Virus, virus rougeoleux.
Molluscum contagiosum Virus	*Molitor hominis, Strongyloplasma hominis.*
Mumps Virus	*Rubula inflans* spec. nov., Virus of epidemic parotis.
Newcastle Disease Virus	*Tortor furens* spec. nov.
Pappataci Fever Virus	Sandfly fever virus.

189

Poliomyelitis Virus	*Legio devilitans,* virus of infantile paralysis, virus poliomyelitique.
Pseudolymphocytic Chorio-meningitis Virus	*Legio simulans* spec. nov.
Rabies Virus	*Formido inexorabilis* spec. nov., street virus, Tollwut-Virus, virus rabique.
Rift Valley Fever Virus	*Charon vallis* spec. nov.
St. Louis Encephalitis Virus	C Encephalitis Virus, *Erro Acelestus.*
Salivary Gland Virus	Cytomegalic inclusion disease virus.
Spring-Summer Encephalitis Virus	*Erro silvestris,* Forest Spring encephalitis virus.
Varicella Virus	*Briareus varicellae,* chickenpox virus.
Variola Virus	*Borreliota variolae,* smallpox virus, *Strongyloplasma variolae.*
Yellow-fever Virus	*Charon evegatus* spec. nov., Gelbfieber-Virus.

REFERENCES

Andrewes, C.H., Chaproniere, D.M., Gompels, A.E.H., Pereira, H.G., and Roden, A.T.: Propagation of common cold virus in tissue cultures. *Lancet, 2:*546, 1953.

Andrewes, C.H.: Adventures among viruses. I. Some properties of viruses. *N Eng J M, 242:*161, 1950.

Andrewes, C.H.: The natural history of the common cold. *Lancet, 1:*71, 1949.

Ayres, J.C., and Feemster, R.F.: Serologic tests in the diagnosis of infectious diseases. *N Eng J M, 243:*996, 1034, 1950.

Babbott, F.L., Jr., and Gordon, J.E.: Modern measles. *Am J Med Sci, 228:* 334, 1954.

Bedson, Samuel, Downie, A.W., MacCallum, F.O., and Stuart-Harris, C.: *Virus and Rickettsial Diseases of Man.* Baltimore, Williams and Wilkins, 1961.

Bland, J.O.W., and Canti, R.G.: The growth and development of psittacosis virus in tissue cultures. *J Pathol Bacteriol, 40:*231, 1935.

Blank, H.: Cytologic smears in the diagnosis of herpes simplex, herpes zoster, and varicella. *J A M A, 146:*1410, 1951.

Boswell, F.W.: Electron microscope studies of virus elementary bodies. *B J Exp Pathol, 28:*253, 1947.

Breed, Robert S., Murray, E.G.D., and Smith, Nathan R.: *Bergey's Manual of Determinative Bacteriology,* 7th ed. Baltimore, Williams and Wilkins, 1957.

Briody, B.A.: Variation in influenza viruses. *Bacteriol Rev, 14:*65, 1950.

Buddingh, C.J., Schrum, D.I., Lancier, J.C., and Guidry, D.J.: Studies of the natural history of herpes simplex infections. *J Pediatr, 11:*595, 1953.

Burnet, F.M.: *Cellular Immunology.* London, Cambridge University Press, 1969.

Busby, D.W.G., House, W., and MacDonald, J.R.: *Virological Technique.* Boston, Little, Brown, 1964.

Casals, J., and Braux, L.V.: Hemagglutination with arthropod-borne viruses. *J Exp Med, 99:*429, 1954.

Cohen, S.M., Gordon, I., Rapp, F., Macaulay, J.C., and Buckley, S.: Fluorescent antibody and complement fixation tests of agents isolated in tissue culture from measles patients. *Proc Soc Exp Biol Med, 90:*118, 1955.

Coons, A.H.: Fluorescent antibodies as histochemical tools. *Fed Proc, 10:* 558-559, 1951.

Christie, A.B.: *Infectious Diseases: Epidemiology and Clinical Practice.* Edinburgh, Livingstone, 1969.

Cunningham, Charles H.: *A Laboratory Guide in Virology,* 6th ed. Minneapolis, Burgess Publishing, 1966.

Dalldorf, Gilbert: *Introduction to Virology.* Springfield, Thomas, 1955.

Dascomb, H.E., Adair, C.V., and Rogers, N.: Serologic investigations of herpes simplex virus infections. *J Lab Clin Med, 46:*1, 1955.

Davidsohn, Israel, and Wells, Benjamin B.: *Clinical Diagnosis by Laboratory Methods.* Philadelphia, W.B. Saunders, 1962.

Denney-Brown, D., Adams, R.D., and Fitzgerald, P.J.: Pathologic features of herpes zoster. *Arch Neurol Psychiatr, 51:*216, 1944.

Diagnostic Procedures for Virus and Rickettsial Diseases, 2nd ed. New York, American Public Health Association, 1956.

Donahue, W.L.: Interstitial plasma cell pneumonia. *Lab Invest, 5:*97, 1956.

Donahue, W.L., Playfair, F.D., and Whitaker, L.: Mumps encephalitis. *J Pediat, 47:*395, 1955.

Downie, A.W., and MacDonald, A.: Smallpox and related virus infections in man. *Br Med Bull, 9:*191, 1953.

Elton, N.W., Romero, A., and Trejos, A.: Clinical pathology of yellow fever. *Am J Clin Pathol., 25:*135, 1955.

Enders, J.F., Peebles, T.C., McCarthy, K., Milovanovic, M.,. Mitus, A., and Holloway, A.: Measles virus: A summary of experiments concerned with isolation, properties, and behavior. *Am J Public Health, 47:*275, 1957.

Erikson, R.L.: Replication of RNA viruses. *Ann Rev Microbiol, 22:*305-322, 1968.

Evans, A.J.: Pathogenicity and immunology of Newcastle disease virus (NDV) in man. *Am J Public Health, 45:*742, 1955.

Fenner, Frank, and White, David: *Medical Virology.* New York, Academic Press, 1970.

Fenner, F.: *The Biology of Animal Viruses.* New York, Academic Press, 1968, Vol. I.

Fowle, A.M.C., Cockeram, A., and Ormsby, H.L.: Virus isolations from patients with keratoconjunctivitis. *Am J Opthalmol, 40:*180, 1955.

Frankel, Sam, Reitman, Stanley, and Sonnenwirth, Alex C.: *Gradwohl's Clinical Laboratory Methods and Diagnosis.* St. Louis, C.V. Mosby, Vol. I, 1963.

Gordon, J.E. (Ed.): *Control of Communicable Diseases in Man,* 12th ed. New York, American Public Health Association, 1969.

Grist, N.R.: *Diagnostic Methods in Clinical Virology.* Philadelphia, F.A. Davis, 1966.

Gross, Ludwik: *Oncogenic Viruses.* Pergamon Press, 1970.

Hampton, A.G., Jr.: Primary varicella pneumonia. *Arch Intern Med, 95:*137, 1955.

Hartman, Frank W., Horsfall, Frank L., and Kidd, John G.: *The Dynamics of Virus and Rickettsial Infections.* New York, Blakison Co., 1954.

Heath, M.D., and Waterson, A.P.: *Modern Trends in Medical Virology.* Butterworths, London, Appleton-Century-Crofts, 1970.

Henle, G., and Deinhardt, F.: Propagation and primary isolation of mumps virus in tissue culture. *Proc Exp Biol Med, 89:*556, 1955.

Hilleman, M.R., Haig, D.A., and Helmold, R.J.: The indirect complement fixation, hemagglutination and conglutinating complement absorption tests for viruses of the psittacosis-lymphogranuloma venereum group. *J Immunol, 66:*115, 1951.

Hilleman, M.R.: Immunological studies of the psittacosis-lympho-granuloma group of viral agents. *J Infect Dis, 76:*96, 1945.

Humphrey, J.H., and White, R.G.: *Immunology for Students of Medicine,* 3rd ed. Oxford, Blackwell, 1970.

Jensen, K.E., and Francis, T., Jr.: The antigenic composition of influenza virus measured by antibody-absorption. *J Exp Med, 98:*619, 1953.

Lazarus, A.S., and Meyer, K.F.: The virus of psittacosis. III. Serological investigation, *J Bacteriol, 38:*171-198, 1939.

Lebrun, J.: Cellular localization of herpes simplex virus by means of fluorescent antibody. *Virology, 2:*496, 1956.

Lennette, E.H., and Schmidt, N.J. (Eds.) : *Diagnostic Procedures for Virology and Rickettsial Infections,* 4th ed. New York, American Public Health Association, 1969.

Lloyd, G.M., Macdonald, A., and Glover, R.E.: Human infection with the virus of contagious pustular dermatitis. *Lancet, 1:*720, 1951.

Low, R.C.: Molluscum contagiosum. *Edinburgh Med J, 53:*657, 1946.

Luria, S.E., and Darnell, J.E.: *General Virology,* 2nd ed. New York, John Wiley and Sons, 1967.

Maramorosch, K.: Friendly viruses. *Sci Am, 203:*138, 1960.

Margileth, A.M.: The diagnosis and treatment of generalized cytomegalic inclusion disease of the newborn. *Pediatrics, 15:*270, 1955.

Meyer, K.F., and Eddie, B.: The knowledge of human virus infections of animal origin. *JAMA, 133:*822, 1947.

Morgan, H.R., and Finland, M.: Serologic findings in patients with primary atypical pneumonia. *Am J Clin Pathol, 18:*593, 1948.

Ormsby, H.L., and Fowle, A.M.C.: Epidemic keratoconjunctivitis. *Am J Ophthalmol, 40:*200, 1955.

Parsons, Rose Morgan, and Schermeister, Leo J.: An indirect hemagglutination test for *Mycoplasma pneumoniae. Am J Med Technol, 34:*453-458, 1968.

Rake, G.: The lymphogranuloma-psittacosis group. *Ann NY Acad Sci, 56:*557, 1953.

Rhodes, A.J., and vanRooyen, C.E.: *Textbook of Virology,* 3rd ed. Baltimore, Williams and Wilkins, 1958.

Rhodes, A.J.: Recent advances in the laboratory diagnosis of virus infections. *Ann Intern Med, 45:*106, 1956.

Rivers, T.M., and Horsfall, F.L.: *Viral and Rickettsial Infections of Man,* 3rd ed. Philadelphia, J.B. Lippincott, 1959.

Sabin, A.B.: Pathogenesis of poliomyelitis. Reappraisal in the light of new data. *Science, 123:*1151, 1956.

Scott, T.F., McN.: Contributions of the virus laboratory to community health. *N Engl J Med, 250:*140, 1951.

Simpson, R.E.H.: Studies on shingles. Is the virus ordinary chickenpox a virus? *Lancet, 2:*1299, 1954.

Smadel, J.E.: The hazard of acquiring virus and rickettsial diseases in the laboratory. *Am J Public Health, 41:*788, 1951.

Smith, W., Andrewes, C.H., and Laidlaw, P.P.: A virus obtained from influenza patients. *Lancet, 2:*66, 1933.

Smithburn, K.C., Haddow, A.J., and Lumsden, W.H.R.: Rift Valley Fever: Transmission of the virus by mosquitoes. *Br J Exp Pathol, 30:*35, 1949.

Stent, Gunther S.: *Papers on Bacterial Viruses.* Berkeley, University of California, 1960.

Tissue Culture and Virus Propagation, 4th ed. Detroit, Difco Laboratories, 1964.

Todd, James Campbell, and Sanford, Arthur Hawley: *Clinical Diagnosis by Laboratory Methods.* Philadelphia, W.B. Saunders, 1943.

VanRooyen, C.E., and Scott, D.G.: Smallpox diagnosis with special reference to electron microscopy. *Can J Public Health, 39:*467, 1948.

VonMagnus, H., Gear, J.H.S., and Paul, J.R.: A recent definition of poliomyelitis viruses. *Virology, 1:*185, 1955.

SECTION IV
RICKETTSIOLOGY

FLEA - BORNE TYPHUS IDENTIFICATION

NURSES' RESPONSIBILITY:

Refer to *Rickettsial Studies, Collection of Specimens,* page 204.

PRINCIPLE OF THE TEST:

This group contains *Rickettsia typhi,* responsible for causing endemic flea-borne typhus. Laboratory identification includes animal inoculation of the patient's blood clot in saline intraperitoneally into guinea pigs. The guinea pigs are observed for swelling ractions of the scrota (Neill-Mooser scrotal reaction) and tunica vaginalis in addition to febrile reactions. Other animals used for studies include rabbits, mice, and rats. Giemsa-stained scrotal tissue may reveal rickettsiae within the endothelial cells of the tunica vaginalis. Serum samples drawn at three days and six days and tested by the Weil-Felix test show a *positive* case of endemic murine typhus as "rise in titer of agglutinins to *B. proteus* OX19." Differentiation of endemic (murine) and epidemic typhus is often made by agglutination and complement-fixation tests of *R. typhi* and *R. prowazekii.* Fluorescent antibody tests are of extreme value.

SPECIMEN REQUIRED:

Ten milliliters of venous blood are withdrawn and allowed to clot, and the serum separated by centrifugation; serum samples are collected at three and six days.

PRESERVATIVE: None required.

LENGTH OF TIME REQUIRED TO PERFORM TEST:
Animal Inoculation: Allow up to two weeks.
Fluorescent Antibody: One to four hours.
Serologic Tests: 24 to 48 hours.

NORMAL VALUES:

No organisms of this group identified by laboratory methods.

POSITIVE IN: Endemic murine flea-borne typhus.

LOUSE - BORNE TYPHUS IDENTIFICATION

NURSES' RESPONSIBILITY:
Refer to *Rickettsial Studies, Collection of Specimens,* page 204.
PRINCIPLE OF THE TEST:

This group of rickettsiae includes those responsible for causing European epidemic louse-borne typhus, Brill's disease (recrudescent epidemic typhus), and trench fever. Laboratory identification of these differ. Each is briefly described.

European Epidemic Louse-Borne Typhus: Isolation of the causal agent, *R. prowazekii,* may be accomplished by injecting an aliquot of the patient's whole blood intraperitoneally into male guinea pigs. After 10 to 12 days and a subsequent temperature rise to 104° to 106°F, the animals are sacrificed and the brain tissue inoculated into embryonated eggs. Serologic tests are also of value. These include the Weil-Felix test, direct agglutination, and completement-fixation tests. Fluorescent antibody tests are of extreme value.

Brill's Disease (Brill-Zinsser Diesase, Recrudescent Epidemic Typhus): Isolation of the causative agent, *R. prowazekii,* has been accomplished by inoculation of the patient's blood intraperitoneally into male guinea pigs or cotton rats during the febrile stage. Hemagglutination and complement-fixation tests are of importance. The Weil-Felix is frequently used but is rarely significant. The fluorescent antibody test is used with extremely good results.

Trench Fever (Werner-His Disease, Polish-Russian Intermittent or Mouse-Fever, Shank Fever, Shin fever): No specific tests are available for trench fever, caused by *R. quintana.* Chick embryo inoculation or animal inoculation are not applicable. The Weil-Felix test is negative. Laboratory diagnosis is frequently accomplished by allowing lice to feed on the patient. Intestinal suspensions of the lice are then inoculated into monkeys, whereby the rickettsiae may be isolated from the monkey's blood. The fluorescent antibody test is used with extremely good results.

SPECIMEN REQUIRED:

European Epidemic Louse-Borne Typhus: Whole blood (untreated), serum (after sixth day for serologic tests.)

Brill's Disease: Whole blood (untreated), serum after third day for serologic tests.

Trench Fever: Serum for serologic tests.

PRESERVATIVE: None required.

LENGTH OF TIME REQUIRED TO PERFORM TEST:

Allow up to 14 days for animal inoculation. Serologic tests—24 to 48 hours.

NORMAL VALUES:

No pathogenic organisms of this group isolated by laboratory methods.

POSITIVE IN: Refer to *Principle of the Test.*

MITE - BORNE TYPHUS IDENTIFICATION

NURSES' RESPONSIBILITY:
Refer to *Rickettsial Studies, Collection of Specimens,* page 204.

PRINCIPLE OF THE TEST:
This group contains the rickettsiae capable of causing tsutsugamushi disease (also known as mite typhus, scrub typhus of Malaya, China fever, Japanese flood fever, and Burma eruptive fever). The causal agent is *R. tsutsugamushi (R. orientalis).*

Laboratory tests for the diagnosis of tsutsugamushi disease include animal inoculation intraperitoneally into albino mice. Smears of the peritoneal exudate, stained with Giemsa's stain, are used to identify any *R. tsutsugamushi* organisms which may be present. The Weil-Felix test is of some value but has been shown to be unreliable in most cases. The fluorescent antibody test is used with good results.

SPECIMEN REQUIRED:
A small aliquot (0.25 ml) of citrated blood, urine, postmortem tissues, serum for Weil-Felix test.

PRESERVATIVE: None required.

LENGTH OF TIME REQUIRED TO PERFORM TEST:
Serologic Tests: 24 to 48 hours.
Animal Inoculation: Allow up to four weeks.

NORMAL VALUES:
No *R. tsutsugamushi* organisms identified by laboratory methods.

POSITIVE IN: Tsutsugamushi disease (scrub typhus).

Q FEVER DIAGNOSTIC TEST

NURSES' RESPONSIBILITY:

Refer to *Rickettsial Studies, Collection of Specimens,* page 204

PRINCIPLE OF THE TEST:

Isolation of the causal agent, *Coxiella burnetii,* may be made by inoculation of the test materials intraperitoneally into guinea pigs, hamsters, and mice. A *positive* fever reaction occurs within five to twelve days. Complement-fixation tests are frequently employed. Egg inoculation is frequently used, employing the yolk sac. Giemsa-stained smears of the infected yolk sac often reveal the *C. burnetii* organisms. The fluorescent antibody test may be used with success.

SPECIMEN REQUIRED:

Clinical specimens include milk, clotted blood, sputum, urine, placental tissues, and postmortem tissues. Serum samples are often collected at the onset of disease and thereafter at intervals of 10 days.

PRESERVATIVE: None required.

NORMAL VALUES: No *C. burnetii* organisms identified by laboratory methods.

LENGTH OF TIME REQUIRED TO PERFORM TEST:

Serologic Tests: 24 to 48 hours.

Animal Inoculation: Allow up to eight weeks.

POSITIVE IN: Q fever.

RICKETTSIAE — NOMENCLATURE

Certain rickettsiae are known to clinicians by various terminology. The following is a listing of the perferred names of the various rickettsiae, as well as some of the most commonly known synonyms.

RICKETTSIAE–PREFERRED NAMES AND SYNONYMS

PREFERRED NAME	SYNONYM(S)
Bartonella bacilliformis	*Bartonia bacilliformis.*
Chlamydia oculogenitalis	*Chlamydozoon oculogenitale,* agent of swimming-pool conjunctivitis.
Chlamydia trachomatis	Agent of trachoma, *Chlamydozoon trachomatis, Rickettsia trachomae, R. trachomatis.*
Coxiella burnetii	Agent of Q fever, *Burnetia (Dyera) burneti, C. diaporica, C. burneti; Rickettsia burneti, R. diaporica.*
Miyagawanella illinii	*Ehrlichia illinii.*
Miyagawanella lymphogranulomatosis	Agent of lympogranuloma venerum; *Chlamydozoon lymphophilus, Ehrlichia lymphogranulomatosis, Rickettsiaformis lymphogranulomatis.*
Miyagawanella ornithosis	Agent of ornithosis, *Chlamydozoon columbi, C. meningophilus, Rickettsiaformis ornithosis.*
Miyagawanella pneumoniae	*Chlamydozoon hominis, Ehrlichia pneumoniae, Rickettsiaformis pneumoniae.*
Miyagawanella psittaci	Agent of psittacosis, *Chlamydozoon psittaci, Ehrlichia psittaci, Microbacterium multiforme psittacosis, Rickettsia psittaci, Rickettsiaformis psittacosis.*
Rickettsia akari	*Acaroxenus varioleidis, Dermacentroxenus akari, Gamasoxenus muris.*

202

Rickettsia conorii	*Dermacentroxenus conori,* *D. pijperi,* *D. rickettsi* var. *conori,* *Ixodoxenus conori, R. blanci,* *R. megawi* var. *pijperi.*
Rickettsia prowazekii	*R. exanthematotyphi,* *R. kairo.*
Rickettsia quintana	*Burnetia (Rocha-Limae) weigli,* *B. (Rocha-Limae) wolhynica,* *R. pediculi, R. weigli,* *R. wolhynica, Wolhynia* *quintanae.*
Rickettsia rickettsii	*Dermacentroxenus rickettsi,* *Ixodoxenus rickettsi, R. brasiliensis,* *R. colombiensis, R. typhi.*
Rickettsia tsutsugamushi	*Dermacentroxenus orientalis,* *R. akamushi, R. megawai* var. *fletcheri,* *R. megawi, R. orientalis,* *R. pseudotyphi, R. sumatranus,* *R. tsutsugamushi-orientalis,* *Theileria tsutsugamushi, Trombiodoxenus orientalis, Zinssera orientalis.*
Rickettsia typhi	*Dermacentoxenus typhi, R. exanthematofebri, R. fletcheri, R. manchuriae,* *R. mooseri, R. muricola, R. murina,* *R. murina mooseri, R. prowazeki* var. *mooseri, R. prowazeki* subsp. *typhi.*

RICKETTSIAL STUDIES

The rickettsiae are organisms which, like the viruses, require both living cells and intracellular enzymes for growth. They occupy a biologic position between the smaller bacteria and the larger viruses. The rickettsiae possess properties of both the viruses and bacteria. They differ from the viruses in that they are capable of proliferating in the intestinal tracts of arthropod vectors. The system of classification of the rickettsiae, like that for the viruses, has been in dispute. Although they are often grouped with the viruses, the rickettsiae more frequently resemble the bacteria. The authors of this book have described the rickettsial identification on the basis of *vectors*. The reader is referred to the individual descriptions of rickettsial diagnoses listed alphabetically as follows:

Flea-Borne Typhus, p. 197.
Louse-Borne Typhus, p. 198.
Mite-Borne Typhus, p. 200.
Q Fever Dignostic Test, p. 201.
Tick-Borne Typhus, p. 206.

Collection of Specimens: The responsibility of the nurse in the collection of specimens for rickettsial studies will vary only slightly. Generally speaking, it is the responsibility of the nurse to assist the physician in obtaining the specimens and to transport these to the laboratory immediately after the collection.

Serological Tests: Numerous serological tests are available for the identification of the rickettsiae. Among these tests are egg inoculation (yolk sac), specific complement-fixation, hemagglutination, fluorescent antibody, and the specific Weil-Felix reaction. With the exception of the Weil-Felix test, these tests are run in the same manner as those for the viruses.

RICKETTSIALPOX IDENTIFICATION

NURSES' RESPONSIBILITY:
Refer to *Rickettsial Studies, Collection of Specimens,* page 204.

PRINCIPLE OF THE TEST:
Isolation of the causal agent, *R. akari,* may be accomplished by inoculation of an aliquot of the patient's blood into albino mice. Chick embryo inoculation and animal inoculation of the guinea pig may also be used. The Weil-Felix test is negative. The complement-fixation test is used with moderate success. The fluorescent antibody test is used with good results.

SPECIMEN REQUIRED:
Paired sera—acute and convalescent—may be used for the complement-fixation and Weil-Felix tests; whole blood is used for animal inoculation.

PRESERVATIVE: None required.

LENGTH OF TIME REQUIRED TO PERFORM TEST:
Serologic Tests: 24 to 48 hours.
Animal Inoculation: Allow up to two weeks.

NORMAL VALUES:
R. akari not isolated or identified by laboratory methods.

POSITIVE IN: Rickettsialpox.

TICK - BORNE TYPHUS IDENTIFICATION

NURSES' RESPONSIBILITY:
Refer to *Rickettsial Studies, Collection of Specimens,* page 204.

PRINCIPLE OF THE TEST:

This group contains rickettsiae responsible for causing Rocky Mountain spotted fever, fever boutonneuse, North Queensland tick typhus, Indian tick typhus, and South African tick-bite fever. Various laboratory tests are available for diagnoses of these diseases. A few representatives of this group are briefly described.

Rocky Mountain Spotted Fever: The causal agent, *R. rickettsii,* may be isolated by inoculating an aliquot of the patient's blood intraperitoneally into male guinea pigs. A positive test reveals edema and ulceration of the scrotum. Endothelial cells, stained by Giemsa's stain, are often found within the endothelial cells. The Weil-Felix test may also be employed, as have agglutination and complement-fixation tests. The fluorescent antibody test is extremely valuable. Neutralization tests are often used.

Fever Boutonneuse: The causal agent, *R. conorii,* may be isolated by inoculating an aliquot of the patient's blood intraperitoneally into male guinea pigs. A positive test reveals an elevated temperature up to 106°F within seven days, and adhesions of the tunica vaginalis as well as scrotal swelling. Giemsa-stained slides often reveal both extra-and intranuclear rickettsiae. The Weil-Felix test and complement-fixation tests may be employed with moderate success. The fluorescent antibody test may be used with moderate success.

North Queensland Tick Typhus: The causal agent, *Ixodes holocyclus,* may be isolated by inoculating an aliquot of the patient's blood intraperitoneally into guinea pigs and mice. After seven days, the mice are sacrificed and the peritoneal exudate observed for the rickettsiae. Guinea pigs infected with the rickettsiae show an elevated temperature up to 106°F and at necropsy show swelling of the tunica vaginalis, marked peritonitis accompanied by fibrinopurulent lesions, and congestion. Giemsa-stained slides may reveal intracytoplasmic rickettsiae. The fluorescent antibody test may be used with moderate success. Neutralization tests may be used.

South African Tick-bite Fever: The causal agent, *R. rickettsia* var. *pijperi,* may be isolated by inoculating a small aliquot of the patient's blood (collected in the febrile stage) peritoneally into male guinea pigs. After infection is evident, the guinea pigs are sacrificed and smears made from the scrotal exudate. Both intranuclear and intracytoplasmic rickettsiae are often found. The Weil-Felix test and complement-fixation test may be employed with moderate success. The fluorescent antibody test may be used with moderate success. Neutralization tests are at times employed.

SPECIMEN REQUIRED:

Serum, blood, sputum, urine, or postmortem tissues may be used.

PRESERVATIVE: None required.

LENGTH OF TIME REQUIRED TO PERFORM TEST:
Serologic Tests: 24 to 48 hours.
Animal Inoculation: Allow up to four weeks.

NORMAL VALUES:

No organisms of the Tick-Borne Fever Typhus group isolated or identified by laboratory methods.

POSITIVE IN: Refer to *Principle of the Test.*

REFERENCES

Bedson, Samuel, Downie, A.W., MacCallum, F.O., and Stuart-Harris, C.: *Virus and Rickettsial Diseases of Man*. Baltimore, William and Wilkins, 1961.

Berge, T.O., and Lennette, E.H.: World distribution of Q fever; human, animal, and arthropod infection. *Am J Hygiene, 57*:125, 1953.

Betts, Alan O.: *Viral and Rickettsial Infections of Animals*. New York, Academic Press, 1969.

Breed, Robert S., Murray, E.G.D., and Smith, Nathan R.: *Bergey's Manual of Determinative Bacteriology*, 7th ed. Baltimore, Williams and Wilkins, 1957.

Derrick, E.H.: The epidemiology of Q fever. A review. *Med J Aust, 1*:245, 1953.

Diagnostic Procedures for Virus and Rickettsial Diseases, 2nd ed. New York, American Public Health Association, 1956.

Felix, A.: Standardization of serological tests for the diagnosis of the typhus group of fevers. *Bull W H O, 2*:637, 1950.

Frankel, Sam, Reitman, Stanley, and Sonnenwirth, Alex C.: *Gradwohl's Clinical Laboratory Methods and Diagnosis*. St. Louis, C.V. Mosby, Vol. I, 1963.

Gear, J.: The rickettsial diseases of Southern Africa. A review of recent studies. *S Afr J Clin Sci, 5*:158, 1954.

Hartman, Frank W., Horsfall, Frank L., and Kidd, John G.: *The Dynamics of Virus and Rickettsial Infections*. New York, Blakiston Company, 1954.

Huebner, R.J.: Rickettsialpox and Q fever. *Bacteriol Rev, 14*:245, 1950. rent knowledge. *Ann Intern Med, 30*:495, 1949.

Huebner, R.J., Jellison, W.L., and Beck, M.D.: Q fever—A review of current knowledge, *Ann Intern Med, 30*:495, 1949.

Lennette, Edwin H., and Schmidt, Nathalie J.: *Diagnostic Procedures for Viral and Rickettsial Infections*, 4th ed. New York, American Public Health Association, 1969.

Lewthwaite, R.: The typhus group of fevers. *Br Med J, 2*:826, 875, 1952.

Lillie, R.D.: *Pathology of Rocky Mountain Spotted Fever. Natl Inst Health Bull*, 177, 1941.

Megaw, J.W.: Scrub typhus as a war disease. *Br Med, 2*:109, 1945.

Murray, E.S.: Brill's Disease. I. Clinical and laboratory diagnosis. *J A M A, 142*:1059, 1950.

Philip, C.B.: Tsutsugamushi disease (scrub typhus) in World War II. *J Parasitol, 34*:169, 1948.

Plotz, H.: North Queensland tick typhus: Studies of the etiological agent and its relation to other rickettsial diseases. *Med J Aust, 2*:263, 1946.

208

Rhodes, Andrew James: *Textbook of Virology,* 5th ed. Baltimore, Williams and Wilkins, 1968.

Rivers, Thomas M., and Horsfall, Frank L.: *Viral and Rickettsial Infections of Man,* 3rd ed. Philadelphia, J.B. Lippincott, 1959.

Smadel, J.E.: The hazard of acquiring virus and rickettsial diseases in the laboratory. *Am J Public Health, 41:*788, 1951.

Todd, James Campbell, and Sanford, Arthur Hawley: *Clinical Diagnosis by Laboratory Methods.* Philadelphia, W.B. Saunders, 1943.

Wolbach, S.B.: Rickettsiae and rickettsial diseases of man: A survey. *Arch Pathol, 50:*612, 1950.

SECTION V
CLINICAL PARASITOLOGY

ARTHROPOD IDENTIFICATION

If the parasite is living, care should be taken to avoid being bitten, since many arthropods transmit diseases. Certain species also may infect a person without actual biting.

The specimen should be placed in a clean receptacle and sent to the laboratory for identification. If no adult parasites are visible, it may be necessary for the physician to scrape the skin from the affected parts.

PRINCIPLE OF THE TEST:

Skin scrapings, or other materials to be used for diagnosis, are placed on a glass slide, and a small amount of aqueous potassium hydroxide is added to clear the specimen. After coverslipping, the slide is examined microscopically for evidence of any parasite in its various stages of maturity. Physical features of the adult species which aid in diagnosis include its size, as well as the number of body segments, legs, antennae, etc. Identification of the egg is made by a well-trained parasitologist.

SPECIMEN REQUIRED: Refer to *Nurses' Responsibility.*

PRESERVATIVE: Alcohol may be used, although none is usually needed.

LENGTH OF TIME REQUIRED TO PERFORM TEST:

A minimum of one hour should be allowed.

SIGNIFICANCE OF FINDINGS:

A few of the diseases transmitted by arthropods are diphyllobothriasis, encephalitis, endemic relapsing fever, epidemic typhus, epidemic relapsing fever, filariasis, malaria, paragonimiasis, plague, Q fever, rickettsialpox, sleeping sickness, spotted fever, trench fever, tularemia, and yellow fever.

A partial listing of the species of arthropods which may be found are *Aedes* (mosquito), *Anopheles* (mosquito), *Ceptus* (harvest mite), *Culex aedes* (mosquito), *Cyclops* (fish louse), *Demodex folliculorum* (follicular mite, mange mite), *Dermacentor andersoni* (Rocky Mountain tick, spotted fever tick),

Glossina (tsetse fly), *Pediculus humanus* var. *capitis* (head louse), *Pediculus humanus* var. *corporis* (body louse), *Phthirus pubis* (crab louse, pubic louse), *Pulex* (flea), *Sarcoptes scabiei* (itch mite), *Trombicula alfreddugesi* (chigger, redbug), *Tunga penetrans* (sand flea).

FLAGELLATES (BLOOD AND TISSUE) IDENTIFICATION

NURSES' RESPONSIBILITY:

It is preferable to obtain a specimen of blood in the interval between 10:00 P.M. and 2:00 A.M., since the parasites are more readily found at that time. Frequently, the physician may deem it possible to perform a spleen, sternal, or liver puncture to obtain the specimen.

PRINCIPLE OF THE TEST:

The two kinds of flagellates of human interest that are found in the blood and tissues are the *Trypanosoma* and the *Leishmania* organisms. The larvae or adult forms of these flagellates may be found on direct microscopic examination of a Giemsa- or Wright-stained blood smear—which has been stained as for a routine differential count. Other methods of diagnosis include culture, animal inoculation, or serologic tests. Examination of a larger quantity of blood is made possible by laking 2 cu mm of capillary blood with dilute acetic acid. Upon complete hemolysis, the tube is centrifuged, the supernatant fluid discarded, and the sediment examined under the microscope. Identification of the organisms depends on size, shape, flagella, nuclei, kinetoplasts, and other specific characteristics. The leishmanial parasites are most often found within the monocytes on the stained blood smear. It is also possible to culture flagellates *in vitro* on rabbit blood agar at room temperature for leptomonal organisms. Bio-assay techniques on mice, guinea pigs, or hamsters may be used, but these procedures are usually not necessary. Tissue biopsies may also be sectioned and examined, and are of prime use in the demonstration of all forms of leishmaniasis and some forms of trypanosomiasis. The chief biopsy material is bone marrow.

SPECIMEN REQUIRED:

A small quantity of capillary blood or tissue biopsy is needed.

PRESERVATIVE:

None is required for blood specimens, which are tested immediately. Tissue specimens are preserved with formalin.

LENGTH OF TIME REQUIRED TO PERFORM TEST:

A minimum of two to four hours should be allowed for the direct smear examination, and two days for the tissue biopsy diagnosis.

NORMAL VALUES: No flagellates found.

SIGNIFICANCE OF FINDINGS:

A few of the most common blood and tissue flagellates, with the diseases resulting from their infestation, are *L. donovani* (visceral leishmaniasis), *L. tropica* (Oriental sore), *L. braziliensis* (mucocutaneous lishmaniasis), *T. gambiense* (African sleeping sickness), *T. rhodiense* (East African sleeping sickness), *T. cruzi* (Chagas' disease).

METAZOA — NOMENCLATURE

Certain metazoa are known to clinicians by various terminology. The following is a listing of the preferred names of the various metazoa, as well as their common names.

METAZOA—PREFERRED NAMES AND COMMON NAMES

PREFERRED NAME	COMMON NAME
Cestodes (Tapeworms)	
Diphyllobothrium latum	Fish tapeworm,
Dipylidium caninum	Dog tapeworm, broad Russian tapeworm.
Echinococcus granulosus	Uniocular hydatid cyst.
Hymenolepis diminuta	Rat Tapeworm.
Hymenolepis nana	Dwarf Tapeworm.
Taenia saginata	Beef tapeworm, unarmed tapeworm.
Taenia solium	Pork tapeworm.
Nematodes (Roundworms)	
Ancylostoma duodenale	Old World hookworm.
Ascaris lumbricoides	Eelworm, roundworm.
Enterobius vermicularis	*Oxyuris vermicularis,* threadworm, pinworm, peatworm.
Necator americanus	American hookworm.
Strongyloides stercoralis	Threadworm.
Toxocara vermicularis	Dog tapeworm.
Trichinella spiralis	Trichina worm.
Trichuris trichiura	Whipworm, *Trichocephalus trichiuris,* *Trichocephalus dispar.*
Trematodes (Flukes)	
Clonorchis sinensis	Chinese liver fluke.
Fasciolopsis buski	Giant intestinal fluke.
Fasciolopsis hepatica	Large liver fluke.
Gastrodiscoides hominis	Intestinal fluke.
Heterophyes heterophyes	Intestinal fluke.
Metagonimus yokogawai	Intestinal fluke.

217

Opisthorchis felineus	Cat liver fluke.
Paragonimus westermani	Oriental lung fluke.
Schistosoma haematobium	Blood fluke.
Schistosoma japonicum	Oriental blood fluke.
Schistosoma mansoni	Liver fluke.

MICROFILARIAE (BLOOD) IDENTIFICATION

NURSES' RESPONSIBILITY:

Diagnosis of the microfilariae is accomplished by demonstration of the parasites by microscopic examination. It is preferable to obtain a specimen of blood between 10 P.M. and 4 A.M. since the parasites are more readily found at that time.

PRINCIPLE OF THE TEST:

Of the five species of microfilariae known to infect man, the three which are of prime human interest are *Wuchereria bancrofti, Brugia malayi,* and *Loa loa.* Other filariae of interest to man include *Mansonella ozzardi* and *Acanthocheilonema perstans.*

The microfilariae (motile embryos) may be found on direct microscopic examination of a Giemsa- or Wright-stained blood smear. A small drop of blood is placed on a slide which is stained as for a routine differential. Other methods of value in the diagnosis of filariasis include skin testing and complement-fixation tests.

SPECIMEN REQUIRED: A small quantity of capillary blood is needed.

PRESERVATIVE: None is required.

LENGTH OF TIME REQUIRED TO PERFORM TEST:

A minimum of two to twenty-four hours should be allowed.

NORMAL VALUES: No microfilariae found.

SIGNIFICANCE OF FINDINGS:

A few of the most common blood microfilariae, with the diseases resulting from their infestation, are *W. bancrofti* (Brancroftian filariasis), *B. malayi* (Malayan filariasis), *L. loa* (loiasis), *A. perstans* (nonpathogenic), *M. ozzardi* (nonpathogenic).

OVA AND PARASITES (FECES) IDENTIFICATION

Synonym: O and P of Stool Specimen.

Synonym: O and P of Stool Specimen.

Nurses' Responsibility:

Proper collection of the fecal specimen is essential in the diagnosis of ova and parasites. To assure passage of a stool sufficiently hydrated to contain the ova or parasites, it is frequently advisable for the patient to have a saline cathartic, such as phospho-soda or sodium sulfate (Glauber's salt). Mineral oils, barium and other such lubricants *must* be avoided.

Physical characteristics of the specimen must be noted and recorded, for this indicates the types of organisms and specimen contains. The surface of the specimen must be searched for macroscopic parasites.

For the diagnosis of *Enterobius vermicularis* (pin worms), a clear cellophane tape technique may be used to obtain the specimen. Pinworms are rarely found in the feces. Since the parasite tends to migrate to the anal orifice during the night, the specimen should be collected from the patient late at night or immediately after he rises in the morning before bathing or defecation. The buttocks are spread, and the sticky side of the tape pressed against the uncleansed perianal area. The adhesive side of the tape is then applied to a microscope slide containing a drop of toluene for microscopic search of the ova.

Fecal specimens collected for other parasites should be collected in a clean container or on clean paper, with transfer to a clean, waxed, cardboard receptacle. The specimen must contain no urine, magnesium, barium, iron, oils, or bismuth salts, since these substances tend to mask certain morphologic characteristics of the specimen. If possible, the entire fecal specimen should be brought to the laboratory or placed in a preservative such as PVA (polyvinyl alcohol) *immediately* after defecation. The laboratory diagnosis of certain diseases caused by parasites will vary; however, the majority of these require a *freshly passed, warm* specimen for examination.

Principle of the Test:

In certain parasitic infestations, either the ova or living parasite will be found in the feces. Several reliable means of identifying these are now in use.

Cellophane Tape Technique: After collection of the specimen, as previously described, the slide is examined under low magnification of the microscope for the presence of the typical *E. vermicularis* ova.

Zinc Sulfate Centrifugal Flotation: This technique is employed for helminth eggs and larvae as well as protozoan cysts. Operculated eggs and those of the schistosomes are not recovered by this means. A small amount of fecal specimen is placed in a tube which is half-filled with tap water, the particles broken up with an applicator stick, and the tube filled to the two-thirds mark with tap water. This procedure is repeated three times, with centrifugation for one minute each at 2300 rpm. The supernatant fluids are discarded each time and a zinc sulfate solution with a specific gravity of 1.18 is added. A platinum loop is used to remove the surface film, which is placed on a coverglass. One drop of iodine solution is added to the coverglass to stain the ova, and the preparation is examined microscopically for ova and cysts.

Formalin-Ether Concentration Test: This method is used chiefly in recovering protozoan cysts and helminth eggs and larvae, although operculated and schistosome eggs are also recovered. The greater portion of the stool specimen is placed in saline and strained through gauze. The specimen is centrifuged at 1500 to 2000 rpm. for two minutes and the supernatant fluid decanted. This step is repeated, after which 10 ml of 10% formalin is added to the sediment, mixed, and allowed to stand for five minutes. Three milliliters of ether are added and the tube shaken vigorously. The tube is centrifuged, with four layers resulting: ether at the top, a plug of debris, formalin solution, and the sediment. The latter is examined both in unstained and iodine-stained smears microscopically.

Wet Mount Technique: This method is used to stain protozoan cysts and tropic forms of amebae and flagellates. A small portion of feces is mixed with a drop of saline on a glass slide, and a drop of dilute iodine solution is added. The coverslipped smear is examined microscopically.

Buffered Methylene Blue Wet Mount Technique: This technique is used in the staining of intestinal protozoa in wet mount preparations. The staining by methylene blue tends to provide a color contrast for easier detection of the organism. A small portion of feces is placed on a slide, and one drop of methylene blue is added. After coverslipping, the preparation is examined microscopically.

Trichrome Technique: A quick and relatively simple method for staining of ova and parasites consists of fixing the material on the slide, running it through several solutions of alcohol, staining with trichrome stain, and counterstaining. The slide is then examined microscopically.

Giemsa Stain: A small portion of feces is placed on a slide and one drop of Giemsa stain added. The slide is cover-slipped and examined microscopically for ova and parasites.

Fluorescent Antibody Technique: Fluorescent antibody techniques are of value in the identification of many parasites, such as the ameba. Refer to page 52 for a complete description of this technique.

SPECIMEN REQUIRED:

A small portion of a freshly passed fecal specimen is usually adequate; however, a 24-hour collection may be required.

PRESERVATIVE:

If the specimen is brought to the laboratory immediately after defecation, no preservative is needed. PVA (polyvinyl alcohol) fixative is an excellent preservative for trophozoites. Either 5% or 10% formalin may be used at times.

LENGTH OF TIME REQUIRED TO PERFORM TEST:

A minimum of two to five hours should be allowed.

NORMAL VALUES:

No pathogenic ova or parasites found. The following protozoa are usually considered nonpathogenic: *Chilomastix mesnili, Endolimax nana, Entamoeba coli, E. polecki* (rarely found in man), *Iodamoeba bütchlii, Trichomonas hominis.*

PATHOLOGICAL FINDINGS:

The following are usually considered pathogenic, although those marked with an asterisk may be asymptomatic:

1. *Protozoa:*

    Amoeba: *Entamoeba histolytica, Dientamoeba fragilis.**

    Flagellates: *Giardia lamblia.**

    Infusoria: *Balantidium coli.**

    Sporozoa: *Isospora hominis.**

2. *Helminths:*

    Cestodes (Tapeworms) : *Diphyllobothrium latum* (fish tapeworm) , *Echinococcus granulosus* (hydatid cyst), *Hymenolepis nana* (dwarf tapeworm) , *Taenia saginata* (beef tapeworm) , *T. solium* (pork tapeworm).

    Nematodes (Roundworms) : *Ancylostoma duodenale* (Old World hookworm), *Ascaris lumbricoides* (roundworm) , *Enterobius vermicularis* (pinworm), *Necator americanus* (American hookworm) , *Strongyloides stercoralis, Trichinella spiralis* (trichina), *Trichuris trichiura* (whipworm) , *Trichostrongylus orientalis, Toxocara vermicularis* (dog roundworm).

    Trematodes (Flukes) : *Clonorchis sinensis** (Chinese liver fluke) , *Fasciolopsis buski* (giant intestinal fluke) , *Fasciolopsis hepatica* (large liver fluke), *Gastrodiscoides hominis* (intestinal fluke) , *Heterophyes heterophyes** (intestinal fluke) , *Metagonimus yokogawai** (intestinal fluke) , *Opisthorchis felineus* (cat liver fluke) , *Paragonimus westermani* (Oriental lung fluke) , *Schistosoma haematobium* (blood fluke) , *S. japonicum* (Oriental blood fluke) , *S. mansoni* (liver fluke) .

PARASITIC SEROLOGICAL TESTS

Although serologic tests for parasites are valued in the diagnosis of parasitic diseases, they are still considered of secondary importance to the actual demonstration of the parasite. Serological tests have been of clinical significance in the following: echinococcosis, kala-azar, toxoplasmosis, and trichinosis. Little value is placed on those performed to verify amebiasis, cutaneous leishmaniasis, filariasis, paragonimiasis, or schistosomiasis.

Serologic tests employ many different methods including ring tests, latex agglutination reactions, complement-fixation, bentonite flocculation, and hemagglutination tests.*

---

*The reader is referred to the following individual parasitic serological tests which are listed alphabetically in the *Serology* section of *Immunohematology Procedures*, another book by the authors (Charles C Thomas, publisher, in press): Brahmachari Test, Cysticercosis Agglutination Test, Formol-Gel Test for Kala-azar, Methylene Blue Test for Toxoplasmosis, Trichinella Bentonite Test, Trichinella Complement-Fixation Test, and Trichinella Latex Agglutination Test.

PROTOZOANS — NOMENCLATURE

Certain protozoans are known to clinicians by various terminology. The following is a listing of the preferred names of the various protozoans, as well as some of the most commonly known synonyms.

PROTOZOANS–PREFERRED NAMES AND SYNONYMS

PREFERRED NAME	SYNONYM(S)
Balantidium coli	*Balantidopsis coli, Balantidium coli, Paramecium coli.*
Entamoeba gingivalis	*E. buccalis.*
Giardia lamblia	*G. intestinalis, Lamblia intestinalis.*
Iodamoeba bütschii	*Endolimax williamsi, I. williamsi.*
Leishmania donovani	*L. canis, L. chagasi, L. infantum.*
Plasmodium falciparum	*Haemamoeba praecox, Laverania malariae, P. immaculatum, P. perniciosum, P. tenue.*
Plasmodium malariae	*Haemamoeba malariae, P. quartanae.*
Plasmodium vivax	*Haemamoeba vivax, P. tertianae.*
Toxoplasma gondii	*T. hominis.*
Trichomonas tenax	*T. buccalis, T. elongata.*
Trypanosoma cruzi	*Schizotrypanum cruzi.*

TRICHOMONAS VAGINALIS TEST

SYNONYM: *T. vaginalis* Test.

NURSES' RESPONSIBILITY:

A small aliquot of vaginal, urethral, or prostatic discharge may be emulsified in a drop of saline placed on a chemically clean slide and coverslipped. The slide must be taken to the laboratory immediately, and must be kept moist to prevent loss of motility. By an alternate procedure, the vaginal swab is placed in a tube containing a small amount of saline to prevent loss of motility.

PRINCIPLE OF THE TEST:

In persistent vaginitis, identification of the protozoan, *T. vaginalis,* is sought. The animal is a large flagellate, actively motile, possessing four anterior whiplike flagella, and an undulating membrane extending one-half to two-thirds of the body. The flagellate may also be demonstrated in the urine, both in men and women, since it is often transmitted by sexual contact. *T. vaginalis* may also be cultured, but this is not a usual procedure when the direct examination reveals it as the causative agent of vaginitis.

SPECIMEN REQUIRED:

A few drops of vaginal discharge of women, or urethral and prostatic discharge of men, are needed.

PRESERVATIVE:

None is permitted, as it tends to kill the organism, thus making the diagnosis extremely difficult.

LENGTH OF TIME REQUIRED TO PERFORM TEST:

A minimum of 15 minutes should be allowed for the direct smear examination.

NORMAL VALUES: No *T. vaginalis* present.

FOUND IN: *Vaginitis* in women, urethritis and prostatitis in men.

REFERENCES

Adams, A.R.D., and Malgraith, B.G.: *Clinical Tropical Diseases.* Springfield, Thomas, 1953.

Belding, D.L.: *Textbook of Parasitology.* New York, Appleton-Century-Crofts, 1965.

Brown, H.W., and Belding, D.L.: *Basic Clinical Parasitology,* 2nd ed. New York, Appleton-Century-Crofts, 1964.

Cahill, K.M.: Echinococcosis. *NY Med, 63*:1964, 1963.

Chandler, Asa C., and Read, Clark P.: *Introduction to Parasitology.* New York, John Wiley and Sons, 1961.

Craig, Charles F., and Faust, Ernest C.: *Clinical Parasitology,* 5th ed. Philadelphia, Lea and Febiger, 1951.

Craig, Charles F.: *Laboratory Diagnosis of Protozoan Diseases.* Philadelphia, Lea and Febiger, 1948.

Dawes, Ben: *Advances in Parasitology.* New York, Academic Press, 1970.

Faust, Ernest C.: *Amebiasis.* Springfield, Thomas, 1954.

Frankel, Sam, Reitman, Stanley, and Sonnenwirth, Alex C.: *Gradwohl's Clinical Laboratory Methods and Diagnosis.* St. Louis, C.V. Mosby, 1963, Vol. II.

Hepler, Opal E.: *Manual of Clinical Laboratory Methods.* Springfield, Thomas, 1962.

Hoare, C.A.: *Medical Protozoology.* Baltimore, Williams and Wilkins, 1950.

Hoogstraal, H.: Ticks in relation to human diseases caused by viruses. *Ann Rev Entomol, 11*:261, 1966.

Kurban, A.K.: Histopathology of cutaneous leishmaniasis. *Arch Dermatol, 93*:396, 1966.

Markell, Edward K., and Voge, Marietta: *Medical Parasitology,* 2nd ed. Philadelphia, W.B. Saunders, 1965.

Miller, Seward E.: *A Textbook of Clinical Pathology.* Baltimore, Williams and Wilkins, 1960.

Moore, D.V.: A review of human infections with the common dog tapeworm, *Dipylidium caninum,* in the United States. *Southwest Vet, 15*:283, 1962.

Morgan, Rose M.: *Guide Questions for Medical Technology Examinations.* Springfield, Thomas, 1966.

Najarian, Haig H.: *Textbook of Medical Parasitology.* Baltimore, Williams and Wilkins, 1967.

Peck, S.M., Wright, W.H., and Gant, J.P.: Cutaneous reactions due to the body louse. *JAMA, 123*:821, 1943.

Pryor, H.B.: *Oxyuris vermicularis.* The most prevalent parasite encountered in the practice of pediatrics. *J Pediatr, 46*:262, 1955.

Russel, B.: Parasitic infestations of the skin. *Practitioner, 195*:621, 1964.

Sawitz, W.G.: *Medical Parasitology.* New York, McGraw-Hill, 1956.

Spencer, Francis M., and Monroe, Lee S.: *The Color Atlas of Intestinal Parasites.* Springfield, Thomas, 1961.

Swartzwelder, J.C.: Clinical ascariasis—An analysis of 202 cases in New Orleans. *Am J Dis Child, 72:*172, 1946.

Todd, James C., and Sanford, Arthur H.: *Clinical Diagnosis by Laboratory Methods.* Philadelphia, W.B. Saunders, 1962.

Vakil, V.V., and Sirsat, M.V.: Cysticercosis in man. *Indian J Med Sci, 19:* 667, 1965.

Watt, L.: Trichomoniasis. *Practitioner, 195:*613, 1965.

Wilmot, A.J.: *Clinical Amoebiasis.* Philadelphia, F.A. Davis, 1962.

GLOSSARY

Acid-fast organism: an organism not easily decolorized by an acid-fast staining method; resistant to decolorization by mineral acid after staining with aniline.

Acquired (disease): one which is not present at birth.

Agar: a gelatinous substance, prepared from seaweed in Japan and India, for use as a base in culture media.

Agar slant: tube of melted agar which is slanted to solidify in order to create a greater surface for bacterial inoculation.

Airborne: carried through the air.

Allantoic cavity: fetal pouch in the embryo of mammals, reptiles, and birds that contributes to the formation of the placenta and umbilical cord.

Amniotic cavity: the inner membrane which envelopes the fetus in the uterus and which produces the amniotic fluid.

Antibiotic: a soluble substance derived from a bacterium or mold that inhibits the growth of other microorganisms.

Antiseptic: a substance that destroys the germs of decomposition, disease, or fermentation.

Arthropod: a segmented invertebrate that has jointed appendages, such as an insect or crayfish.

Aseptic: pertaining to a condition in which living pathogenic organisms are absent.

Atomize: to reduce a fluid to the form of a spray.

Autogenous: self-produced; term applied to vaccines or toxins; manufactured from the cultures of patients, for the purpose of therapy for the same patient.

Autopsy: an internal examination of a deceased person, performed to determine the cause of death.

Bacillus (pleural—bacilli): a bacterium that is rod-shaped.

Bacterium (pleural—bacteria): a one-celled microorganism commonly known as a "germ."

Benzidine: para-diamino-diphenyl; used as a test for the identification of occult blood.

Bronchial cast: a cast that originates in the bronchioles.

Broth: a fluid medium used for bacterial growth.

Budding: an outgrowth of small protuberances; may be said of yeast cells which exhibit such characteristics.

Cestode: a tapeworm.

Chorioallantoic membrane: extraembryonic membrane, in bird embryos; formed by the joining of the allantois (respiratory organ) with the serosa or false chorion.

Chromogen: a microorganism capable of producing pigment.

"Clock-streak" method of bacterial isolation: a method of bacterial streaking whereby the original material is thinned out in a clocklike motion.

Coliform: pertaining to the colon bacillus.

Colony: a clone or group of cells or bacteria, growing in a culture media, each the result of multiplication of an individual cell.

Contaminate: to touch with an infectious material.

Culture: the growth of microorganisms in or on artificial media.

Curschmann's spirals: spiraled masses of mucus that occur in the sputum of patients suffering from bronchial asthma.

Decapsulate: removal of the renal capsule.

Differential plate media: a media which contains substances used for a specific purpose, such as isolation and/or identification of a particular microorganism.

Disinfectant: an agent which destroys bacteria.

Dittrich's plugs: masses found in the sputum of patients suffering from gangrene of the lungs or septic bronchitis.

Duodenal: pertaining to the duodenum.

Dysfunction: abnormal function.

Elastic fibers (sputum): elastic fibers of pulmonary substance that are found in destructive diseases of the lung, such as advanced cases of tuberculosis.

Embryo: the initial developing stage of an organism, from one week after conception to the end of the second month.

Feces: waste matter, such as food residues and bacteria, that is discharged from the intestines.

Fermentation: chemical process of decomposition of an organic compound which is brought about by a ferment.

Filaria: a slender, threadlike worm; a nematode that may be found as a parasite in blood or tissues of vertebrates.

Filarial: pertaining to or caused by filariae.

Fungi: a phylum of plants lacking chlorophyll or other pigments necessary for photosynthesis, which live either in or on living or dead organic matter.

Gamete: a germ cell (ovum or sperm) ; refers to the malarial parasite, either a male form (microgamete) or female (macrogamete) .

Gametocyte: the mother cell of a gamete.

Gastric lavage: washing out of the stomach by abundant injections and rejections of water.

Graafian follicle: a vesicular body in the ovary, which contains the ova.

Gram-negative: an organism that loses the crystal violet stain by decolorization with ethanol-acetone but stains with the counterstain of safranin when stained by the Gram staining procedure.

Gram-positive: an organism that retains the crystal violet stain when stained by the Gram staining procedure.

Guaiac: a resinous substance used for the testing of occult blood in various clinical materials.

Helminth: a wormlike parasite which inhabits the intestine.

Host: the organism in which a parasite lives.

Infusion agar: a culture media used in the isolation of microorganisms.

Infusoria: a ciliated class of Protozoa. The members have a generative micronucleus and a vegetative macronucleus.

Inoculate: to introduce material, suspected of containing microorganisms, into culture media.

Inoculum: material introduced by inoculation.

Intermediate host: that which hosts a parasitic protozoan during completion of the asexual cycle.

Invertebrate: lacing a spiral or vertebral column.

Irradiate: to shed light upon a structure or organism.

Isolate: to set apart; detach.

Isolation media: media used to obtain pure cultures of bacteria.

Latent: referring to a period of the disease in which it is not notably active.

Lecithin: a complex yellowish-brown fatty substance that is prepared from the yolk of egg by abstraction with alcohol; insoluble in water; soluble in fatty oils and absolute alcohol.

Liquefaction: the process of making liquid.

Lyophilize: freeze-dry; to separate a solid substance from a solution.

Mammal: a member of the class of vertebrates, *Mammalia*, whose young feed upon milk from the mother's breast.

Media: material in/on which bacteria and/or other microscopic organisms may be grown for cultural characteristics.

Metabolism: the sum of the processes by which an organism uses food for protoplasm and energy production, for storage, and for elimination of waste.

Metastasize: to invade or spread by metastasis.

Metastasis: transition of carcinoma cells from one part of the body to another.

Microbiology: the study of microscopic organisms, such as bacteria.

Microorganism: an organism, of plant or animal origin, that is of microscopic or submicroscopic size.

Microscopic: an object so minute that it can be seen only with the aid of a microscope.

Mite: a minute, parasitic animal, related to the spider, and capable of transmitting disease organisms; a member of the order Acarina.

Motility: the movement of microorganisms.

Mucopurulent: containing both mucus and pus.

Mucosa: a mucous membrane.

Mutation: a variation in a strain, which appears suddenly, due to a change in the gene (s) .

Mycelium: threadlike filaments that constitute the fungus.

Mycology: the study of fungus (i) .

Myxovirus: a name given to the viruses of the influenza group.

Nasopharynx: the part of the pharynx which lies above the soft palate.

Necrosis: death of living tissue.

Nematode: a class of helminths that consist of roundworms, hookworms, pinworms, and whipworms.

Nonpathogenic: not producing or causing disease.

Nutrient agar (broth): a bacterial culture medium consisting of an aqueous solution of beef extract and peptone.

Occult blood: concealed or hidden blood; in a form not readily recognized.

Output: metabolic waste products eliminated from the body.

Ova: plural form of ovum, which is an egg or female sexual cell.

Parasite: a plant or animal that lives upon or within another, and at whose expense it derives its nourishment.

Pathogenic: causing disease.

Pellicle: a surface film or membranelike scum which may be found in fluids, especially those with a high protein content, or as a surface growth in a nutrient broth.

Penicillinase: an enzyme which prevents the antibacterial action of penicillin.

Petri dish: a round shallow dish with cover, used for culturing bacteria and fungi.

Phage: bacteriophage; a viral agent which causes transmissable dissolution of specific bacteria.

Phagocytosis: process whereby foreign substances and microorganisms are ingested and digested by cells.

P.P.D.: abbreviation for purified protein derivative, an extract from tubercle bacilli.

P.P.L.O.: mycoplasma; abbreviation for pleuropneumonia-like organisms.

Protozoa: a phylum of the animal kingdom which consists of all unicellular forms, and of which there are four classes.

Pulmonary function: relating to the capacity and activity of the lungs.

Purulent: containing or forming pus.

Putrefaction: act or process of rotting.

Quellung reaction: differential typing of pneumococci, based on the capsular swelling in the presence of its homologous serum.

Rickettsia: a small, gram-negative, pleomorphic organism that stains well with Giemsa stain; an obligate parasite found intracellularly in arthropods and rodents, transmitted to man by arthropod vectors.

R.N.A.: abbreviation for ribonucleic acid.

Rodent: a gnawing or nibbling animal, such as a beaver or squirrel.

Satellite: a minor structure accompanying a major structure, such as a colony of one organism growing more rapidly near a colony of another organism, or an appendage of a chromosome.

Schüffner's dots (granules, punctation): granules appearing in red blood cells of patients infected with the malarial parasite, *Plasmodium vivax.*

Selective media: bacterial culture media which contains substances that inhibit the growth of certain organisms, while enhancing (permitting) growth of others.

Sensitivity study (bacterial): a test procedure in which discs impregnated with various antibiotics are planted on a plate inoculated with a patient's bacterial culture, to determine which antibiotics will inhibit the growth of the bacteria.

Sensitize: to make cells or bacteria into a condition in which they may be destroyed by the action of substance such as complement.

Serial dilutions: dilutions of serum, with the concentration of serum per diluent being decreased 50 percent in each consecutive tube.

Species: one type of microorganism; a subdivision of genus.

Spirochaete: a spiral-shaped bacterium, such as *Treponema pallidum,* the causative agent of syphilis.

Spore: reproductive cell of a sporozoan or fungus, which is capable of growing directly into a new organism.

Sporozoa: a class of Protozoa that possesses no locomotive organs and reproduce primarily by the formation of spores.

Sputum: a mucoid substance that is expectorated in lung disease.

Stab culture: a technique for inoculating media by piercing the tube of media to the bottom, with the platinum needle coated with the infectious material.

Stabile: firm or steady; not moving; does not disintegrate readily

Strain (bacterial): a pure culture of bacteria, each having a specific designation, such as *Escherichia coli.*

Streak culture: a technique for inoculating media by smearing the surface of the tube or plate of media with a platinum loop or cotton swab coated with the infectious material.

Tapeworm: an intestinal parasite, *Taenia.*

T.B.: abbreviation for tubercle bacillus.

Tenacity: cohesiveness; stickiness.

Transudate: a substance that has passed through a membrane, such as sweat through the skin.

Trematode: a class of helminths that are flukes.

Undulating membrane: a locomotor organ (membrane), projecting laterally from various one-celled organisms; particularly well formed in trypanosomes.

Vector: a "carrier" which transfers an infective agent from one host to another.

Viable: the condition of living and growing.

Viral: referring to virus.

Virologist: a person who studies any virus, or virus-producing disease.

Virology: the study of virus disease.

Virulent: referring to a microorganism which has the ability to produce disease.

Virus: a submicroscopic or ultramicroscopic microorganism, characterized by a lack of metabolism, and capable of producing disease in the presence of living host cells, tissue medium, or developing chick embryo.

Yeasts: fungal microorganisms.

Zone of inhibition: in a bacterial sensitivity study, the area surrounding antibiotic discs which have prevented growth of microorganisms.